Kailin Gow's Go Girl Guide to

the Perfect Cup to Healthy Smoothies and Juices

GUIDE AND RECIPES for BUSY PEOPLE ON THE GO

KAILIN GOW

Kailin Gow

Kailin Gow's Go Girl to the Perfect Cup:
Healthy Smoothies and Juices
Published by Sparklesoup Inc.
Copyright © 2024 Kailin Gow

For information, please contact:

Sparklesoup Inc.
11700 W. Charleston Blvd. #170-95
Las Vegas, NV 89135
www.sparklesoup.com
First Edition.
Printed in the United States of America.

DEDICATION

To my family and friends for encouraging me to write books I believe in. And to my fans for being the best cheerleaders, beta testers, and super fans an author can dream of.

Kailin Gow

Table of Content

The A to Z of Superfoods to Use in Smoothies and Juices

Best Cancer Prevention Superfoods Smoothies and Juices

Best Antioxidant Superfoods Smoothies and Juices

Best Blood Pressure Superfoods Smoothies and Juices

Best Superfoods to Fight or Prevent Diabetes Smoothies and Juices

Best Superfoods for Joints and Arthritis Pain Smoothies and Juices

Best Superfoods to Build Muscles Smoothies and Juices

Best Superfoods to Build Bones Smoothies and Juices

Best Superfoods to Build Blood Cells Smoothies and Juices

Best Superfoods to Get You Going Smoothies and Juices

Best Superfoods to Help Keep Your Guts and Kidneys Healthy Smoothies and Juices

Recipes for Smoothies and Juices Using the Superfoods List

Introduction

What's so Super about Superfoods and Why We Should Consider Consuming Them as Smoothies or Juices?

Super foods are the superheroes amongst foods which have the power to help fight or prevent diseases, keep you healthy and strong, and or provide more energy.

Some boast the power to help you lose weight, maintain your youth and beauty, and even reverse aging.

These foods are no ordinary foods, but have the extra or superpowers to help you be super and keep on the go so you can accomplish super awesome feats!

Some can be found in your everyday grocery stores, while others are rarer, and have to be found online or at specialty stores. Some have been known to be foods we eat every day to stay healthy while others are now becoming known to the general public about being a super healthy food. We've compiled lists of Superfoods here in this guide along with their superpowers.

Additionally, we've compiled easy to tear out lists of Superfoods who are the Best in fighting or preventing certain diseases. Lastly, eating these superfoods must be pleasurable so we've added a large cookbook section on recipes containing these superfoods such as smoothies or juices.

Why Should We Consume Superfoods as Smoothies or Juices?

1. A nutritious and compact way to get more of your daily fiber, vitamins, fruit, vegetables, and superfoods intake.
2. Easier on your stomach and gut.
3. Easy to prepare.
4. Quick to prepare.
5. Portable for the Busy person on the go!

Hopefully with more knowledge about the foods you choose to eat, you can take better care of your body, your health, and always be ready to get ready set and go! Below are the superfoods and their superpower to help you get started, and as with any diet, always consult with your dietitian or physician before embarking on a new diet, especially if you have restrictions.

A to Z

ACAI BERRIES

High in Anthocyanin which power boosts antioxidants in your blood cells.

AGAR

Made of seaweed, it contains calcium, fiber, and iron. It is also used to detoxify.

ALMONDS

High in Vitamin E which heals wounds and build scar tissue. Also helps promote collagen.

APPLES

High in Quercetin which boosts antioxidants and reduce lung cancer.

APRICOT

High in Fiber and Vitamin A.

ARTICHOKE HEARTS

Helps lower cholesterol.

ARUGULA

High in Nitrates which prevent muscle fatigue by improving oxygen delivery to muscles, and arugula dishes up more than any other green. Also good for bone and heart health.

ASPARAGUS

High in Vitamin K and folate to build bones. Also is a diuretic to banish bloating.

AVOCADO

High in good fats that helps you absorb other nutrients. Also good for your skin and hair. Helps promote collagen.

BAKED POTATO

High in Potassium which lowers blood pressure.

BANANAS

High in Fiber, Potassium, and starch to help you slim down and have energy power. Good for better sleep, heart health, and digestion.

BARLEY

High in Beta-glucan which lowers cholesterol and helps control blood pressure.

BARLEY TEA

Popular in Asia, this drink is sold in cans in vending machines but also can be brewed like a tea. Used as a digestif and contains antioxidants.

BEANS

High in Iron which builds new blood cells.

BEETS

Contains vitamins and minerals to help fight off cancer and other diseases and strengthen organs.

BELL PEPPERS

High in Vitamin C which is good for weight loss and building a stronger immune system.

BLACK BEANS

High in antioxidants like protein, fiber, flavoids. Fights Type 2 Diabetes and protects against cancer.

BLACKBERRIES

Have more antioxidants than strawberries, cranberries, and blueberries.

BLUEBERRIES

Brain food that improves memory and reduces inflammation in the brain. Help promote collagen.

BOK CHOY

High in Calcium which helps build bone density and also helps regulate mood swings.

BRAN FLAKES

High in Fiber to keep your heart healthy and melt away belly fat.

BRAZIL NUTS

High in Selennium.

BROCCOLI SPROUTS

High in glucoraphanin.

BROWN RICE

High in Magnesium mineral which helps our body chemicals work together to build bones, mend tissues, and keep the blood flowing. High in fiber to keep you energized longer.

BRUSSEL SPROUTS

High in Glucosinolates which helps combat cancer and detoxify the body.

BUCKWHEAT SOBA NOODLES

High in Magnesium and helps fight Type 2 Diabetes, good for digestion, heart health, and promotes sleep.

CABBAGE

Highly nutritious, cabbage helps boost overall health. Good for eyesight, fight cancer, lower cholesterol, and promote good skin.

CANTALOPE

Acts as a diuretics to rid the body of excess water and waste from the kidneys to relieve stomach bloat. Packs 120% of your recommended daily allowance (RDA) of Vitamin A as well as a whopping 108% of your RDA of Vitamin C per cup. Also it is good for your skin. Good for collagen production for the skin.

CARROT

Good for eyesight and full of fiber. Good source of Thiamin, Niacin, Vitamin B6, Folate and Manganese, and a very good source of dietary fiber, Vitamin A, Vitamin C, Vitamin K and Potassium.

CAULIFLOWER

High in Glucosinolates which helps fight and prevent cancer.

CELERY

Acts as a diuretic to rid the body of excess water and waste from the kidneys to relieve stomach bloat.

CHERRY TART DRINK

High in melatonin, a hormone that helps regulate your sleep cycle. Also good for Gout relief, preventing metabolic syndrome, easing sore muscles.

CHIA SEEDS

High in Protein and Omega-3s for healthier heart and muscle building. Also helps with dry eyes.

CHILI POWDER

High in capsinoids, which burn belly fat.

CINNAMON

Helps keep diabetes at bay and also helps protect heart and improve memory.

CITRUS FRUITS

High in Vitamin C which repair collagen and tissue.

COFFEE

Contains polyphenols which helps the heart and improves memory.

COLLARD GREENS

High in Lutein, Vitamin A, and Zeaxanthin which keeps your eyes healthy.

COCONUT

Contains medium chain triglycerides that may boost metabolism. Also known to rehydrate dry skin and hair.

DARK CHOCOLATE

Protect the heart and improves memory.

DRIED TART CHERRIES

High in potent anthrocyanins which controls blood sugar, lower cholesterol, and reduce insulin.

EGGS

High in Protein that gives you energy and low in calories. Eggs helps keep you energized while slimming you down.

EDAMAME

High in Fiber, Folate, and Phytosterols which lowers cholesterol.

EXTRA VIRGIN OLIVE OIL

High in polyphenols protect brain cells from free radicals that lead to memory loss. Also good for cancer protection and heart health.

FENNEL

Acts as a diuretics to rid the body of excess water and waste from the kidneys to relieve stomach bloat.

FLAXSEEDS

Highest in lignans to prevent ovarian and endometrial cancers. Also has fiber and heart-healthy Omega-3s fat.

GARLIC

Helps prevent heart disease and inflammation. Also helps fight cartilage damage and Arthritis.

GINGER

Natural pain reliever and heart health promoter. Also helps build immunity, intestinal health, cancer protection, and Arthritis.

GOJI BERRIES

Long used in Chinese medicine, the Goji Berries have diabetes and cancer-fighting antioxidants. They have Vitamin A which is good for the skin and eyes, and Vitamin C and Selenium.

GRAPES

High in heart-healthy resveratrol a plant chemical that sweeps Alzheimers-inducing beta-amyloid plaques from the brain. Also good for heart and causes sleep.

GRAPEFRUIT

High in naringenin, which may help burn fat.

GREEK YOGURT

Higher in protein than regular yogurt.

HONEY DEW

Acts as a diuretics to rid the body of excess water and waste from the kidneys to relieve stomach bloat.

HOT PEPPERS

Promotes better digestion, an improved immune system. and better blood circulation and digestion. There is even a rumor that hot peppers aid in weight loss by increasing your metabolism.

JUJUBE

Tastes like apples and eaten in Asia, the jujube fruit helps relieves stress and contains antioxidants.

KABUCHA MELON

The Japanese squash can be a substitute for pumpkin but has few calories and more antioxidants. Also has beta-carotene for beautiful hair and skin.

KALE

High in Carotenoids to fight sun damage. Helps build collagen for good skin and joints.

KEFIR

Packs more probiotic than yogurt so this tangy drink is good for your gut. Also good for cancer protection, fatigue, and PMS.

KIMCHI

Is a traditional Korean dish of fermented spicy cabbage. It is full of probiotics which fights bad bacteria in the body.

KIWI FRUIT

Has 110% Vitamin C Daily Requirement. Good for the heart, offer a host of important vitamins and nutrients, and can even help fight inflammation and cancer.

KONJAC ROOT

Full of fiber, it also has blood pressure lowering potassium and bone building calcium.

LEMON AND LIME

High in loaded with antioxidants, packed with Vitamin C, and offer fabulous benefits to the digestive and respiratory systems.

LENTIL

High in protein, folate, and Vitamin B.

MAITAKE MUSHROOMS

Helps prevent cancer, build immune system, lower blood pressure.

MANGO

Loaded with fiber, potassium, Vitamins A, C, and E, healthy enzymes and antioxidants. Studies show that mangoes are helpful in aiding digestion, maintaining a healthy blood pressure and heart rate, and lowering bad cholesterol levels. In addition, these yummy summer staples have been known to protect against colon, breast, prostate, and leukemia cancers. The combination of certain vitamins and antioxidants make mangoes effective in keeping the skin clear and healthy, too. Also, mangos can be used as an aphrodisiac.

MILK
Ultimate energy drink filled with protein, Vitamin D, and Calcium.

MUNG BEAN SPROUTS
Contains Vitamins B, C, folate, and iron. This sprout can be used in soups, salads, sandwiches or stir fry.

MUSHROOMS
High in Vitamin D which helps heal bones.

MUSTARD GREENS
High in Vitamin K and helps build collagen.

NECTARINES
High in fiber, betacarotene, and Vitamin A for more energy and better vision.

NONFAT RICOTTA CHEESE

From whey protein, ricotta can enhance muscle building and metabolism.

NORI

Dried Seaweed is used in sushi that contains iodine. Good for metabolism, thyroid, blood Stevia regulation, heart health and weight loss.

OLIVES

High in good fats which keeps your heart healthy.

ORANGES

Provides 100% Vitamin C, and also calcium and folate. Suppress appetites because of the pectin it contains. Oranges contain antioxidants to help in the fight against free radicals and prevent signs of aging. Recent research also suggests that oranges contain a natural skin cancer-fighting element. In addition, oranges contain a large number of plant-based chemicals that give protection to the cells and prevent age-related illnesses.

PAPAYA

Papaya contains many superpowers including fighting heart disease, preventing cancer, improving digestion, good for eyes, and protect skin.

PEACHES

High in Fiber to keep you feeling full longer, Vitamin C for better immune system,

PEANUT BUTTER

High in Arginine, an amino acid that helps regulate blood vessels. Also helps lower insulin sensitivity which helps reduce the risk of diabetes.

PEARS

High in Flavonoids which helps reduce risk of heart disease and fiber to keep you feeling full longer.

PINEAPPLE

Bromelain breaks down protein to aid in digestion and can also be useful as an anti-inflammatory. Bromelain has been shown to be useful in treating acute sinusitis, arthritis, gout, sore throats, as well as gastrointestinal issues. High in antioxidants, keep eyes healthy, and increase energy.

PISTACHIO

High in protein, potassium, and fiber.

POMEGRANITE

High in Vitamin C to prevent skin damage and premature aging. Also has punicalagin which fights against the breakdown of collagen, preserving joint health.

POPCORN

High in fiber and polyphenols which contaiantioxidants.

POULTRY

High in rotein to repair tissues.

PUMPKINS

High in alpha and beta-carotene which helps fight and prevent cancer.

PUMPKIN SEEDS

High in magnesium, a mineral that helps muscles (and your rattled nerves) relax. Also good for controlling blood sug control and heart health.

PRUNES (DRIED PLUMS)

High in Polyphenols which helps build blood cells and bone density.

QUINOA

Full of fiber to help you have energy and steady blood Stevia level. Good for weight loss, heart health, and protection against ulcers.

RASPBERRIES

High in Fiber and Vitamin C which is great for the immune system.

RED ONIONS

Full of anti-inflammatories and antioxidants to protect against heart disease, cancers, and ulcers.

ROMAINE LETTUCE

Full of vitamin A, plus 113% of bone-building vitamin K.

SAUERKRAUT

Full of fiber which gives you energy and probiotics which fights bad bacteria in the belly.

SEAFOOD

High in Zinc which gives energy and heals tissues.

SEAWEED SOUP

Eaten in Asia, it is high in calcium, Omega-3s, vitamins and minerals that it is used to nourish pregnant women.

SALMON

High in Omega 3s to keep your heart healthy.

SHITAKE MUSHROOMS
High in Vitamin D.

SOY MILK
High in Vegetable Protein, Calcium, and Vitamin D. Also help produce collagen which is good for the skin and joints.

SPINACH
High in Vitamin K which builds strong bones and prevent blood clots.

SPIRULINA
Contain protein content will help your muscles stay strong and repair themselves after difficult workouts. Also contains Vitamin B to help build blood cells.

STEEL-CUT OATS
High in Fiber which keeps you full and energized longer.

STRAWBERRY
High in phytochemicals and ellagitannins which helps halt the growth of cervical and colon cancer.

SWEET POTATOES

High in Vitamin A which helps build the immune system, promote cell growth, and protect vision.

SUNFLOWER SEEDS

Has half the daily requirements for Vitamin E to keep your skin smooth, heart healthy, and fights infection.

TARO

Is like an Asian Potato and has many nutrients such as Potassium, iron, zinc, Vitamin B6, Vitamin C, fiber, and even protein.

TEA (BLACK AND GREEN)

Prevent hardening of arteries, promotes healing from sun damage, acts as an antioxidant, and help prevent skin cancer. Green tea also helps fight dementia and promotes metabolism.

TOMATOES

High in Lycopene which makes your skin look younger and heart healthier.

TUNA

High in Protein and Selenium which promotes elastin which keeps skin smoother and tight.

TURKEY BREAST

High in Protein but low in calories.

TURMERIC

Keeps the mind young by preventing Alzheimers.

UNSWEETENED COCOA

High in flavonols which relax arteries and reduce blood pressure. Also good for insulin regulation and brain health.

VINEGAR

Vinegar has been shown to have antioxidant and antibacterial properties. Vinegar has also been shown to help control blood pressure and blood Stevia, assist with weight loss by increasing satiety after meal. Best use in moderation.

WALNUTS

High in Alpha-linolenic Acid and Omega-3 fat to help improve memory and concentration.

WATER

Water provides hydration which minimizes fatigue and dizziness.

WATERCRESS

High in Vitamin K, Lutein, Beta-Carotene, and Phytochemicals so it is good for vision and fights cancers.

WATERMELON

High in water which keeps you hydrated and feeling full. Also contains lycopene which helps prevent sun damage.

WHEAT GERM

High in Vitamin E and Selenium to boost immune system.

WHOLE WHEAT ENGLISH MUFFINS

High in Fiber but low in calories for more energy.

WHOLE GRAINS

High in Fiber to regulate bowel movement to prevent constipation.

YAKULT

A yogurt-like drink filled with Probiotics which is a staple daily drink in Asia.

YOGURT

High in Calcium and Probiotics which regulates the gastrointestinal system.

Mix in Blueberries and flaxseeds for better skin.

ZUCCHINI

High in pectins which promotes heart health and lowers cholesterols.

Kailin Gow

Best Cancer Prevention Superfoods

Tomatoes
Watermelon
Cabbage
Carrots
Pasta
Bean
Broccoli
Peppers
Dried Apricots
Sunflower Seeds
Blueberries
Strawberries
Chocolate
Goji Berries
Acai Berries
Green Tea
Turmeric
Pistachios
Garlic
Brussels Sprouts
Cabbage

Coffee
Curry
Farmed Rainbow Trout
Grapes
Kiwifruit
Mushrooms
Onions
Oregano
Peanuts
Pumpkin Seeds
Skimmed Milk
Tart Cherries

Kailin Gow

Best Antioxidant Superfoods

Bilberries
Black Currants
Strawberries
Cranberries
Ground Clove
Peppermint
Allspice
Cinnamon
Oregano
Thyme
Sage
Rosemary
Saffron
Basil
Chives
Dill
Parsley
Walnuts
Pecans
Chestnuts
Almonds
Hazelnuts

Sunflower Seeds
Espresso
Coffee
Green and Black Tea
Pomegrante Juice
Grape Juice
Red Wine
Artichokes
Curly Kale
Red and Green Chili Peppers
Red Cabbage
Red Beets
Dark Chocolate
Apples
Goji Berries
Acai Berries

Kailin Gow

Best Superfoods to Lower Blood Pressure

Kale
Broccoli
Beets
Red Bell Pepper
Peaches and Nectarines
Bananas
Kiwifruit
Blueberries
Tomatoes
Lemons
Fat-free Plain Yogurt
Tilapia
Pork Tenderloins
White Beans
Extra-Virgin Olive Oil
Vitamin K2
Green Tea
Green Coffee
Turmeric
Fish Oil
Cashews and Almonds

Garlic

Kailin Gow

Best Superfoods to Fight or Prevent Diabetes

Dark Chocolate
Broccoli
Blueberries
Steel-cut Oats
Fish
Olive Oil
Psyllium husk
Cannellini Beans
Walnuts
Quinoa
Cinnamon
Turmeric
Spinach
Sweet Potatoes
Collard Greens

Best Superfoods for Joints and Pain Relief

Blueberries
Strawberries
Citrus fruit
Kale
Spinach
Red peppers
Carrots
Cherries
Salmon or mackerel
Nutmeg
Ginger
Cayenne
Oregano
Flaxseeds
Hemp seeds or oil
Walnuts
Avocados
Olive oil
Garlic
Leeks
Onions

Apples
Almonds
Chia
Purslane
Sacha inchi oil
Pineapple
Bromelain
Papaya
Extra Virgin Olive Oil
Coconut Oil
Red Bell Pepper
Bananas
Avocado
Turmeric
Ginger
Kale

Best Superfoods to Build Bones

Yogurt
Milk
Salmon and Tuna
Other Fish
Lean meats
Fortified Foods
Spinach
Greek Yogurt
Eggs
Nut Butter

Kailin Gow

Best Superfoods to Build More Blood Cells

Spinach
Turnips Greens
Legumes
Whole Grains
Raisins
Blackstrap Molasses
Pumpkin Seeds
Other Seeds
Cereals
Bread
Iron-Fortified Flour
Fish
Long-grain Rice
Turkey
Chicken
Potatoes
Bananas
Whole Grains
Nuts
Beef liver
Fish

Red Meat
Eggs
Milk
Dairy Products
Long-grain Rice
Turkey
Chicken Giblets
Asparagus
Broccoli
Brussels Sprouts
Lettuce
Dark Leafy Greens

Kailin Gow

Best Superfoods for Energy to Get You Going

Flaxseeds
Avocado
Tomatoes
Yogurt
Kale
Almonds
Walnuts
Olive Oil
Turmeric
Hemp Protein Powder
Dried Fruits
Rosemary
Leeks
Figs
Carrots or Carrot Juice
Mushrooms
Kiwi
Quinoa
Salmon
Acai

Virgin Coconut Oil

Kailin Gow

Best Superfoods for Keeping Your Kidneys and Gut Healthy

Cabbage
Watercrest
Cauliflower
Leafy greens
Dandelion greens
Spinach
Cucumbers
Radish
Cilantros
Celery
Carrots
Sweet Potatoes
Bok Choy
Red bell peppers
Berries, especially raspberries
Pomegranate
Black plums
Apricots
Cherries
Cranberries
Grapes
Peach
Pear

Pineapples
Plums
Tangerines
Oranges
Eggplants
Fig
Mustard Greens
Okra
Onions
Radicchio
Rhubarb
Turnips
Water chestnuts
Watermelon
Legumes and Beans, especially green beans
Melons
Apples
Bananas
Lemons
Coconuts
Ginger with Thyme
Turmeric
Black pepper
Unsalted nuts
Rice
Barley

Kailin Gow

Air-popped popcorn
Polenta
Yogurt
Green tea
Beet juice
Seltzer water
Apple Cider Vinegar

Superfoods Pairings

Combine Superfoods for an easier and more flavorful meal or snack. Here are a few ways to combine superfoods:

• Salad with mandarin oranges and toasted slivered almonds

• Spinach salad with orange slices

• Oatmeal with strawberries

These can be eaten as is or blended with ice and your favorite liquid such as water, seltzer water, juice, tea, rice or almond milk into a smoothie.

Kailin Gow

Creating Your Own Smoothies to Fit Your Special Diet Needs

Now that you have a list of foods for each special diet, you can get creative in making your own special smoothies or juice.

You can basically make smoothies out of any of these foods by adding, combining them with the liquid of your choice (water, juice, tea, milk, etc.) with sweeteners (honey, monkfruit, molasses, stevia, etc.) and without to make healthy and delicious smoothies every day. The following are some recipes to help you get started!

Recipes for Smoothies

APPLE AND PEACH SMOOTHIE

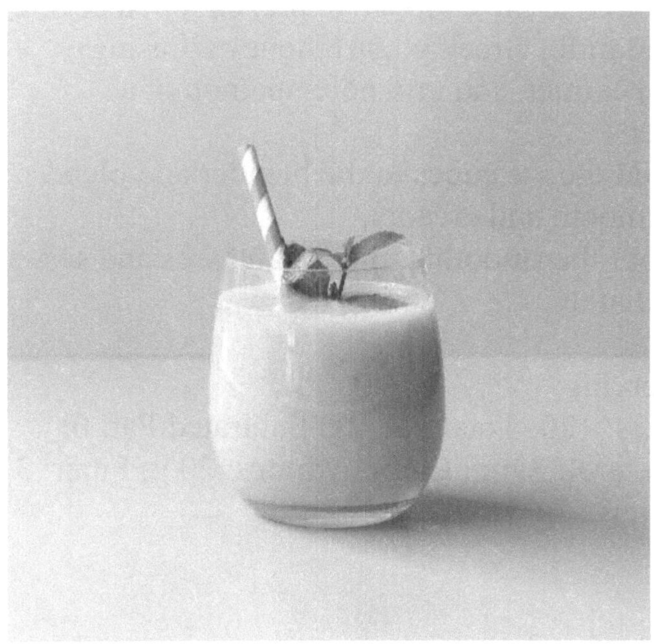

Prep Time: 10 Minutes
- 1 medium apple, cored and chopped
- 1 ripe peach, peeled and chopped

- ½ cup unsweetened almond milk
- ½ cup plain low-fat Greek yogurt
- 1 teaspoon honey
- ½ teaspoon vanilla extract
- 12 teaspoon ground cinnamon
- 1 cup ice cubes

Instructions:

1.   Combine the chopped apple, chopped peach, almond milk, Greek yogurt, honey (if using), vanilla extract, and ground cinnamon in a blender.
2.   Add the ice cubes to the blender and blend until smooth and creamy.
3.   Pour the smoothie into two glasses and serve immediately.

Per Serving:
Calories: 120: Total Fat: 2g: Saturated Fat: 0g: Cholesterol: 3 mg; Carbohydrates: 20 g; Fiber: 3 g; Protein: 7g

CRANBERRY SMOOTHIE

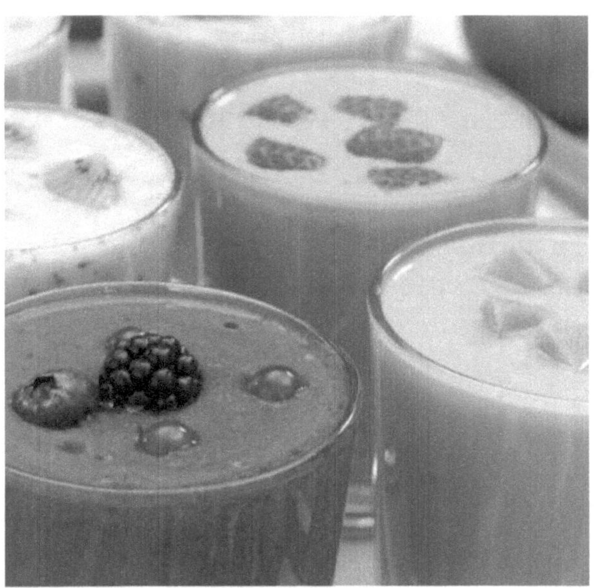

Prep Time:
- 1 cup unsweetened cranberry juice
- ½ cup frozen cranberries
- ½ cup low-fat plain yogurt
- 1 tablespoon honey (optional)
- 1ce cubes

Instructions:

1. Combine the cranberry juice, frozen cranberries, low-fat plain yogurt, and honey (if using) in a blender.
2. Add a few ice cubes to the blender and blend until smooth.
3. Adjust the sweetness with more honey if needed.
4. Pour the smoothie into two glasses and serve immediately.

Per Serving: Calories: 110; Total Fat: 1 g; Saturated Fat: 0 g: Cholesterol: 2 mg; Carbohydrates: 23 g; Fiber: 2 g: Protein: 3 g; Phosphorus: 60 mg: Potassium: 290 mg.

BERRY BREEZE SMOOTHIE

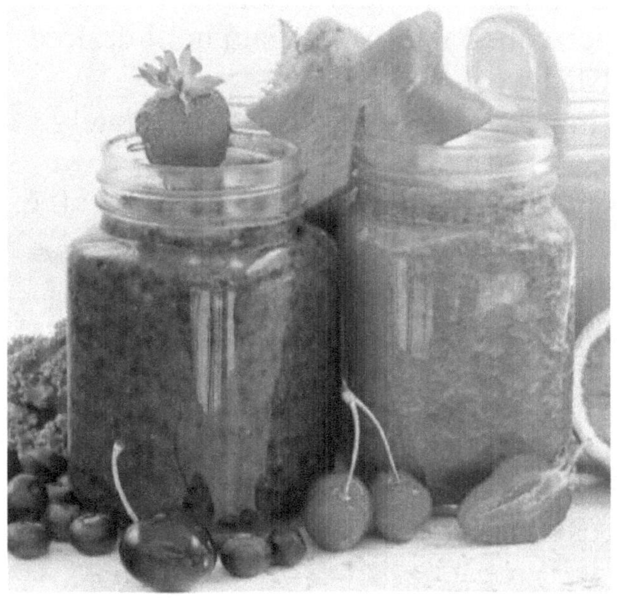

Prep Time: 5 minutes

- ½ cup raspberries
- ½ cup strawberries
- 1 cup unsweetened almond milk
- ¼ cup low-fat Greek yogurt (unflavored)
- 1 tablespoon honey
- ½ teaspoon vanilla extract

- 1 cup ice cubes

1. Combine raspberries, strawberries, almond milk, Greek yogurt, honey, and vanilla extract in a blender.
2. Blend until smooth and creamy.
3. Add ice cubes and blend again until desired consistency.
4. Pour into 2 glasses and serve immediately.

Calories: 123; Total Fat: 2g: Saturated Fat: 0 g: Cholesterol: 0 mg: Carbohydrates: 23 g: Fiber: 4 g: Protein: 5 g: Phosphorus: 100 mg: Potassium: 210 mg: Sodium: 85 mg

PINEAPPLE APPLE SMOOTHIE

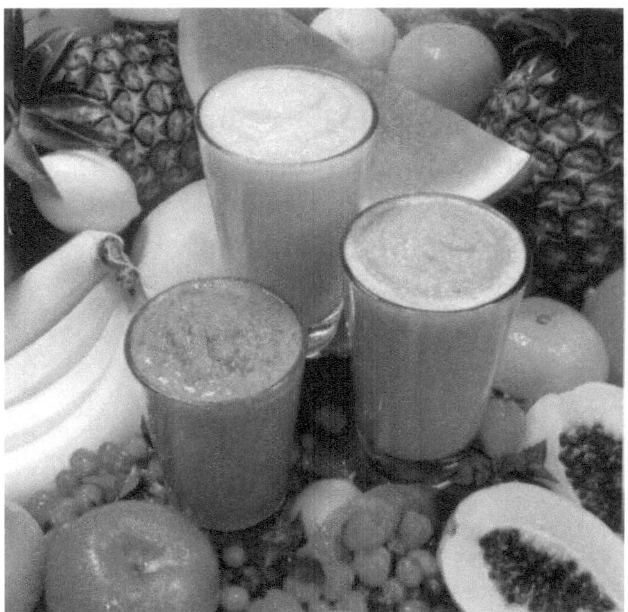

Prep Time: 10 Minutes

- 1 cup fresh pineapple, cubed
- 1 medium apple, peeled, cored, and chopped
- 1 cup unsweetened almond milk
- ¼ cup crushed ice
- 1 tablespoon honey

- ½ teaspoon ground cinnamon

In a blender, combine pineapple, apple, almond milk, crushed ice, honey and cinnamon

Blend until smooth and creamy.

Pour into 2 glasses and serve immediately.

Calories: 160: Total Fat: 3 g: Saturated Fat: 0 g: Cholesterol: 0 mg: Carbohydrates: 34 g: Fiber: 4 g: Protein: 2 g: Phosphorus: 57 mg: Potassium: 286 mg: Sodium: 86 mg

CUCUMBER MELON SMOOTHIE

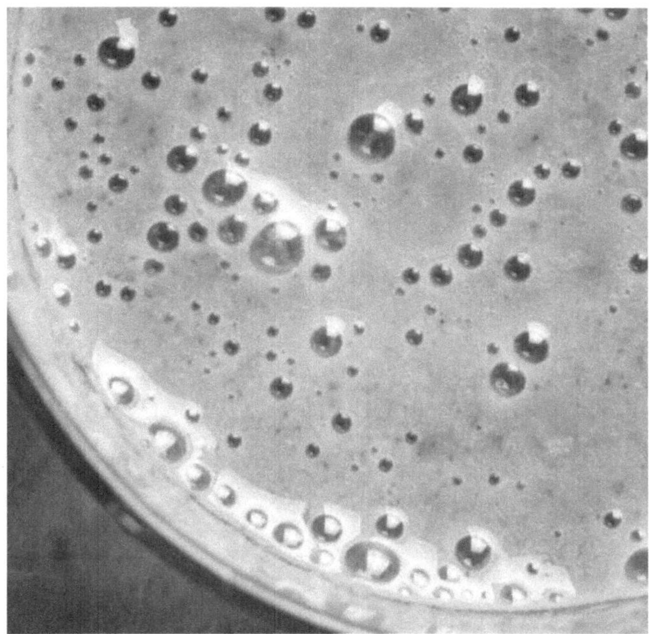

Prep Time: 10 Minutes

- 1 cup honeydew melon, cubed
- ½ cup cucumber, peeled and chopped
- 1 cup unsweetened coconut water
- 1 tablespoon fresh mint leaves
- 1 tablespoon lemon juice

- 1 cup ice cubes

In a blender, combine honeydew melon, cucumber, coconut water, mint leaves, and lemon juice.

Blend until smooth and creamy.

Add ice cubes and blend again until desired consistency is reached.

Pour into 2 glasses and serve immediately.

Calories: 78: Total Fat: 0 g: Saturated Fat: 0 g: Cholesterol: 0 mg: Carbohdrates: 19 g: Fiber: 2 g: Protein: 1 g: Phosphorus: 35 mg: Potassium: 250 mg: Sodium 98 mg.

BANANA STRAWBERRY CHIA HONEY SMOOTHIE

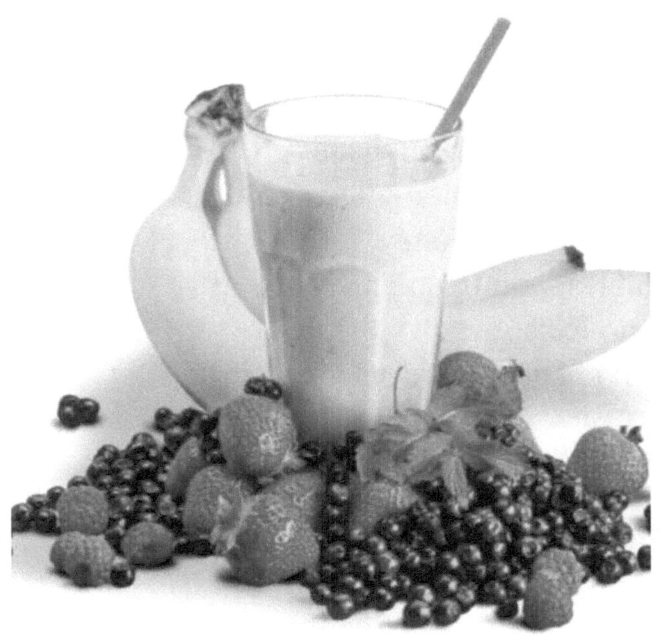

- 1/2 cup strawberries, frozen
- 1/2 cup sliced bananas, frozen
- 1/2 cup kefir or Greek yogurt
- 1 tablespoon chia seeds
- 1/2 cup almond milk, unsweetened
- splash of vanilla extract
- 1 tablespoon honey

Place all ingredients in a blender and blend until smooth! Let sit for a few minutes until chia seeds expand and enjoy.

LEMON GINGER SPARKLING WATER

- 1 ½ cups sparkling water
- ½ cup fresh lemon juice
- 2 tablespoons honey
- 1 tablespoon fresh giner, grated
- 1 cup ice cubes
- Lemon slices and fresh mint leaves for garnish

In a small bowl, combine lemon juice, honey, and grated ginger. Stir well.

Fill 2 glasses with ice and the mixture evenly.

Garnish with lemon slices and fresh mint leaves optional.

Calories: 70: Total Fat: 0 g: Cholesterol: 19 g

CARROT MANGO SMOOTHIE

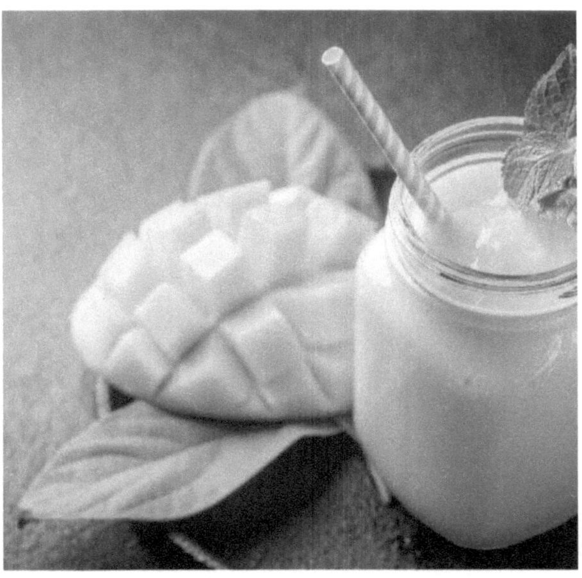

- 1 cup carrots, peeled and chopped
- 1 cup fresh mango, cubed
- 1 cup unsweetened almond milk
- ¼ cp low-fat Greek unflavored yogurt
- 1 tablespoon honey
- ½ teaspoon ground ginger
- 1 cup ice cubes

In a blender, combine carrots, mango, almond milk, Greek yogurt, honey, and ground ginger.

Blend until smooth and creamy.

Add ice cubes and blend until desired consistency.

BLUEBERRY PEACH SMOOTHIE

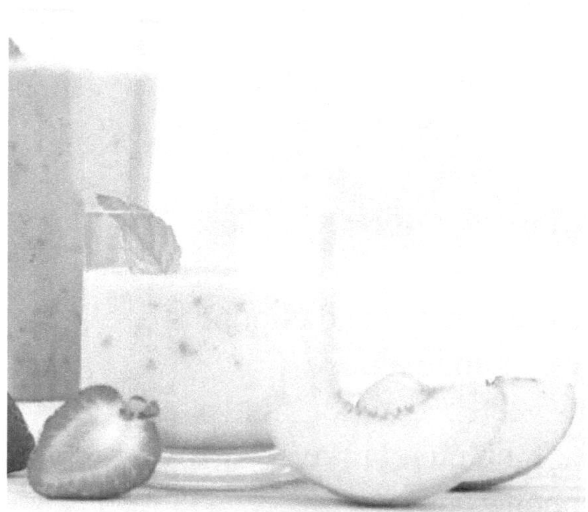

- 1 cup fresh blueberries
- 1 medium peach, pitted and chopped
- 1 cup unsweetened almond milk
- ¼ low-fat Greek unflavored yogurt

- 1 tablespoon honey
- 1 teaspoon vanilla extract
- 1 cup ice cubes

In a blender, combine blueberries, peach, almond milk, Greek yogurt, honey, and vanilla extract.

Blend until smooth and creamy.

Add ice cubes and blend until desired consistency.

GREEN GRAPE SMOOTHIE

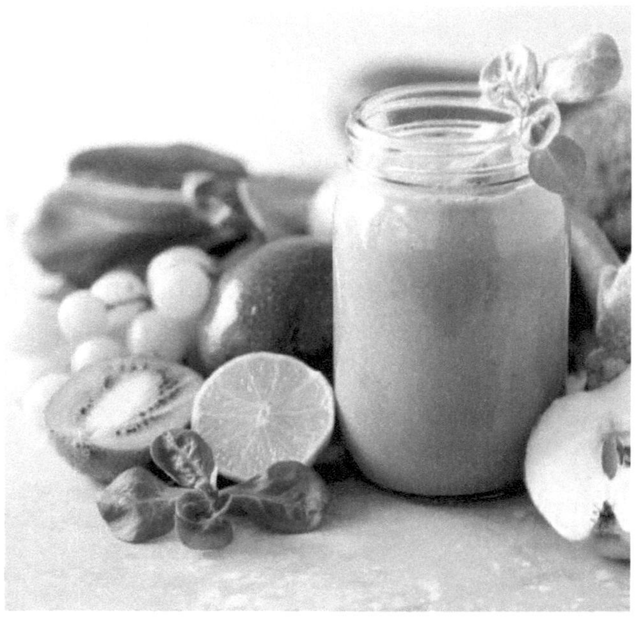

- 1 ½ cups green grapes
- ½ medium cucumber, peeled, and chopped
- 1 cup unsweetened almond milk
- ½ cup ice cubes
- 1 tablespoon honey
- Fresh mint leaves for garnish

In a blender, combine green grapes, cucumber, almond milk, ice cubes, and honey.

Blend until smooth and creamy.

Pour into 2 glasses, garnish with fresh mint leaves.

Kailin Gow

CHERRY VANILLA SMOOTHIE

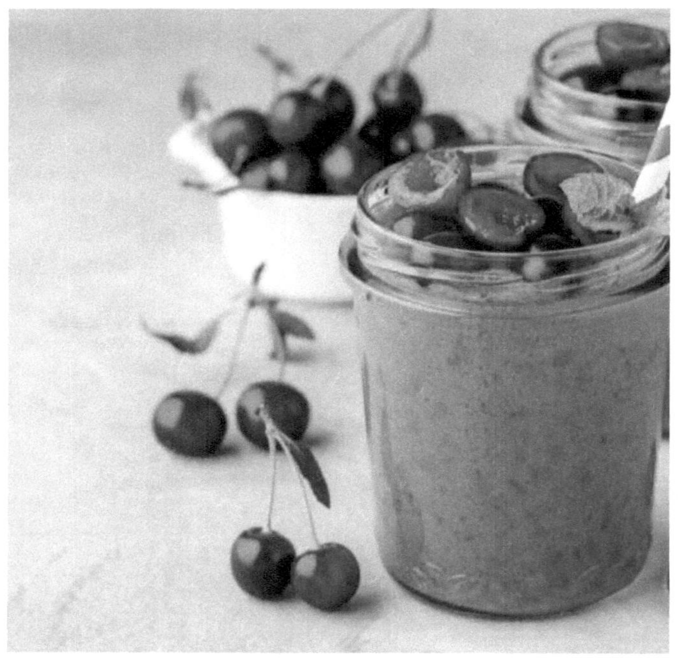

- 1 cup fresh cherries pitted
- 1 cup unsweetened almond milk
- ½ cup low-fat ricotta cheese
- 1 tablespoon honey
- 1 teaspoon vanilla extract
- 1 cup ice cubes

In a blender, combine cherries, almond milk, ricotta cheese, honey, and vanilla extract.

Blend until smooth and creamy.

Add ice cubes and blend again until desired consistency.

BERRY GREEN SMOOTHIE

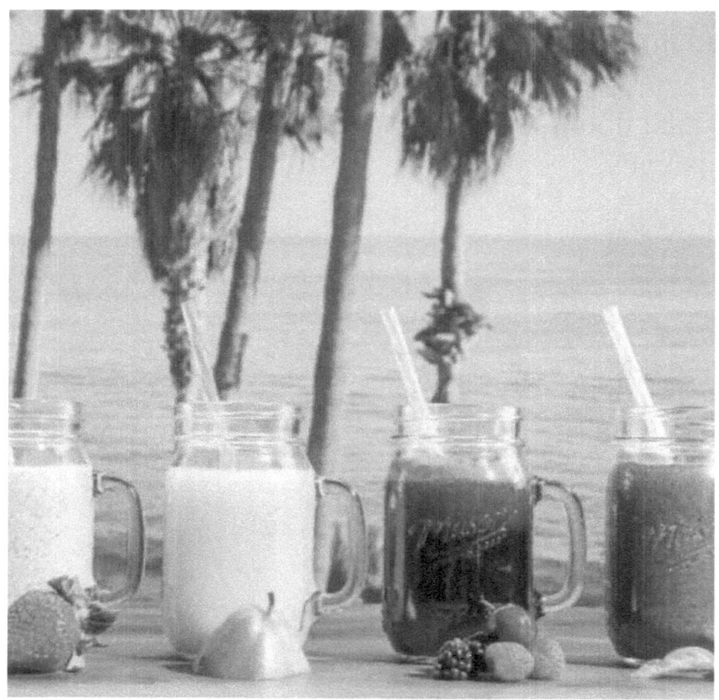

- 1 cup frozen blueberries or mixed berries
- ½ cup fresh baby spinach leaves
- 2 tablespoons fresh orange juice
- 2 tablespoons water
- 1 5.3 ounce plain 2% Greek yogurt or plain soy yogurt

- 1 sliced medium ripe banana

Put all the ingredients into a blender and blend until smooth. Serve immediately.

CHERRY POWER SMOOTHIE

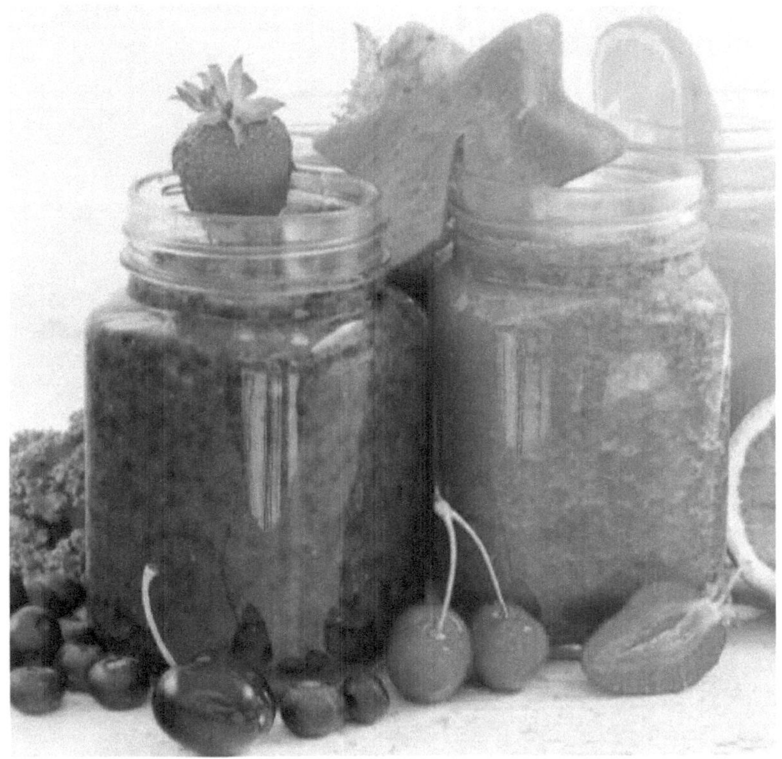

- 1 small ripe banana
- 1 ½ cups frozen pitted dark sweet cherries
- ½ cup plain 2% Greek yogurt or drained soft tofu
- 1/3 2% milk or unsweetened nondairy milk
- 1 tablespoon fresh lemon juice
- 2 teaspoons ground flaxseed
- 2 teaspoons honey, or ½ teaspoon liquid stevia

Place all ingredients into a blender, blend until smooth and serve immediately.

DARK CHOCOLATE SMOOTHIE

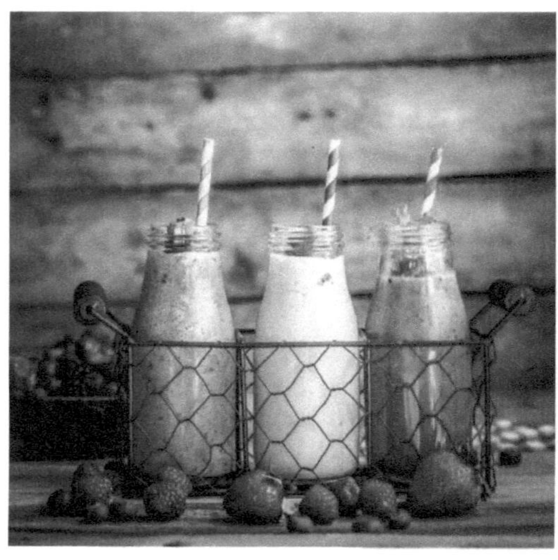

- 3 pitted dates
- 1 cup unsweetened chocolate almond milk
- 1 cup ice
- 1 tablespoon unsweetened cocoa powder
- 1 (5.3 ounce) container vanilla soy yogurt
- ½ banana, sliced and frozen
- (Optional) Dash of instant coffee

Soften the dried dates in a small bowl of hot water for 3 minutes.

Place the milk and dates in a blender and blend for 30 seconds until pureed. Add the ice, cocoa powder, yogurt, banana, and coffee and blend until smooth.

Kailin Gow

WATERMELON CUCUMBER SMOOTHIE

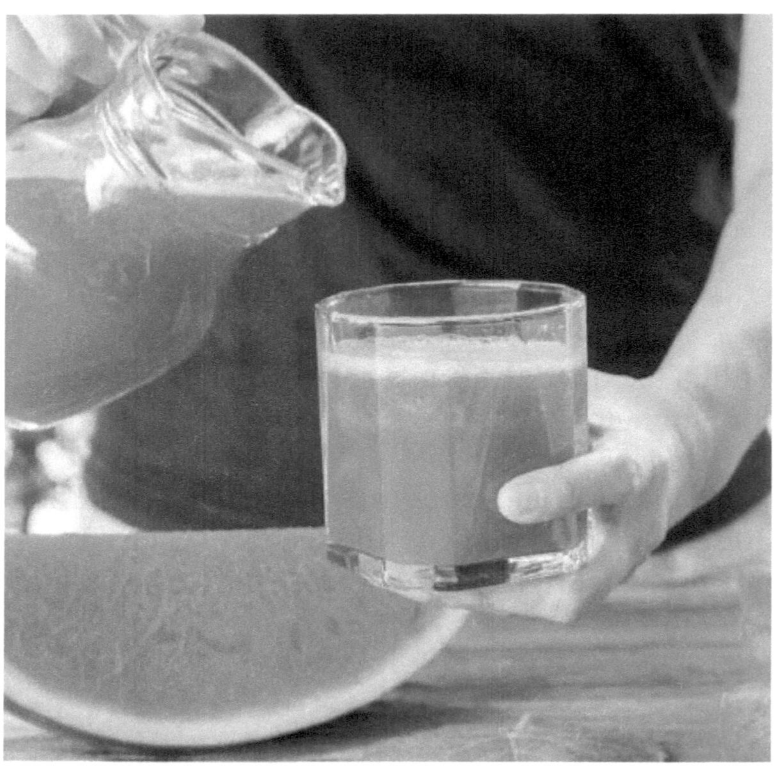

- 2 cups chopped watermelon
- 1 medium peeled and sliced cucumber
- 2 sprigs of mint (use only the leaves)
- 1 celery stalk
- Ice
- Squeeze of lime

Blend all ingredients in a blender until creamy.

APPLE BANANA SMOOTHIE

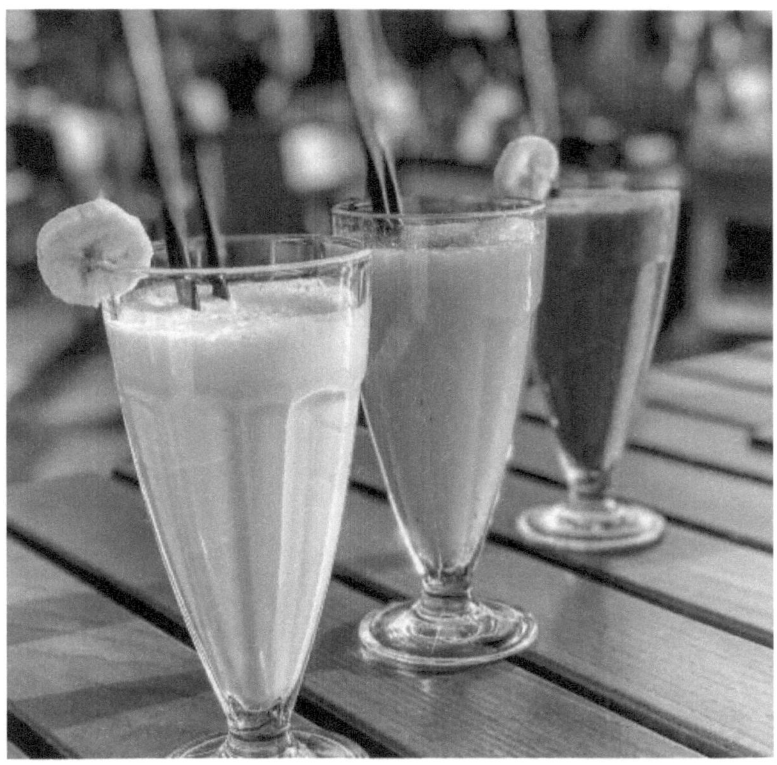

- ½ a banana
- ½ cup plain yogurt
- ½ cup apple sauce
- ¼ cup almond or rice milk

- 1 tbsp honey
- Ice (optional)

Blend all ingredients in a blender until creamy.

TROPICAL FRUIT SMOOTHIE

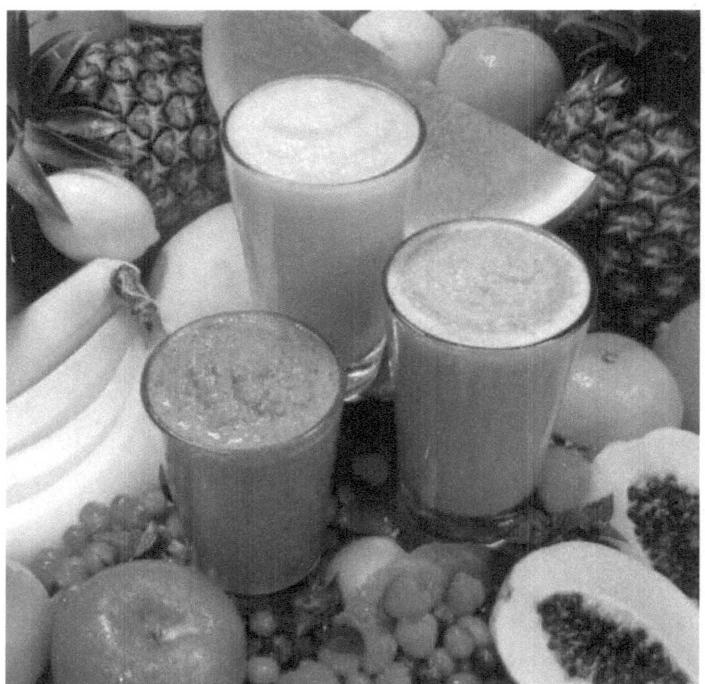

- ½ cup pineapples
- ½ cup strawberries
- 1 small orange, peeled
- ½ cup rice milk
- Ice

Blend all ingredients in a blender until creamy.

RASPBERRY PEACH SMOOTHIE

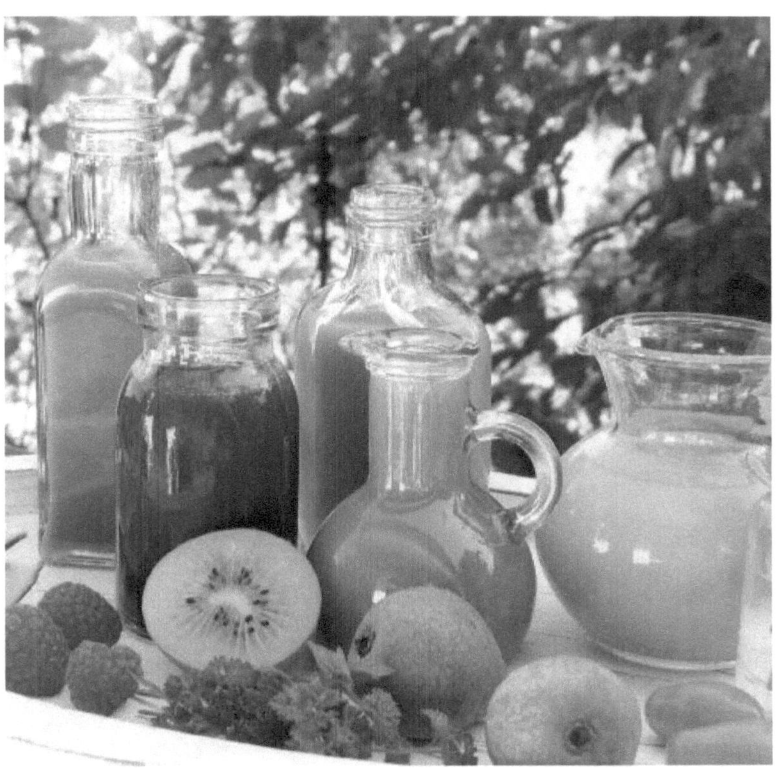

- ½ cup frozen peaches
- 1 cup frozen raspberries
- ½ cup soft tofu

- 1 cup vanilla flavored almond milk
- 1 tbsp honey

Blend all ingredients in a blender until creamy.

RED, WHITE, BLUEBERRIES SMOOTHIE

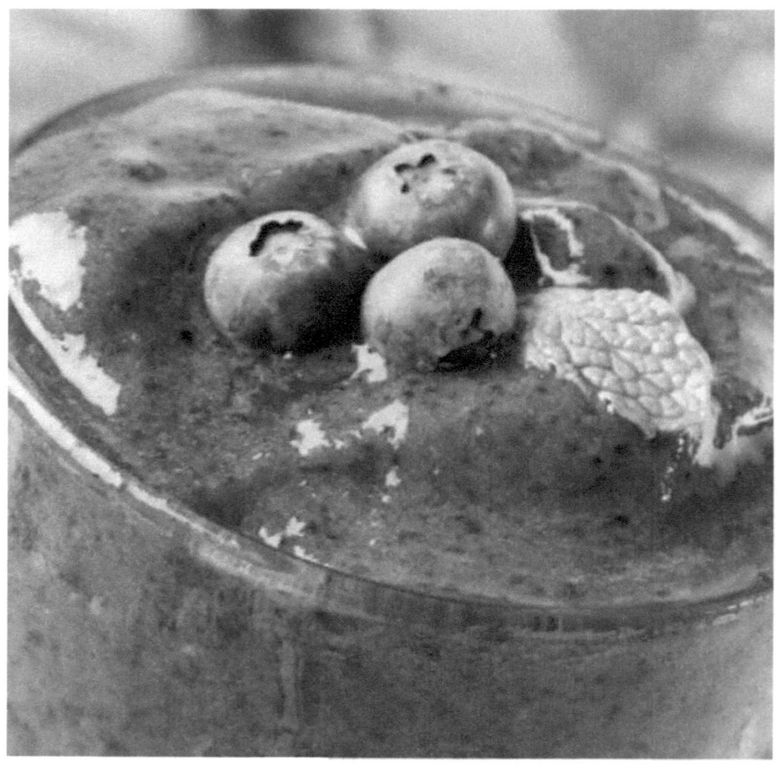

- ½ cup frozen unsweetened raspberries
- ¼ cup unsweetened cranberry juice

- ½ cup frozen unsweetened blueberries
- 2/3 cup silken firm tofu
- 1 tsp vanilla extract
- Ice (optional)

Blend all ingredients in a blender until creamy.

POMEGRANATE RADICCHIO SMOOTHIE

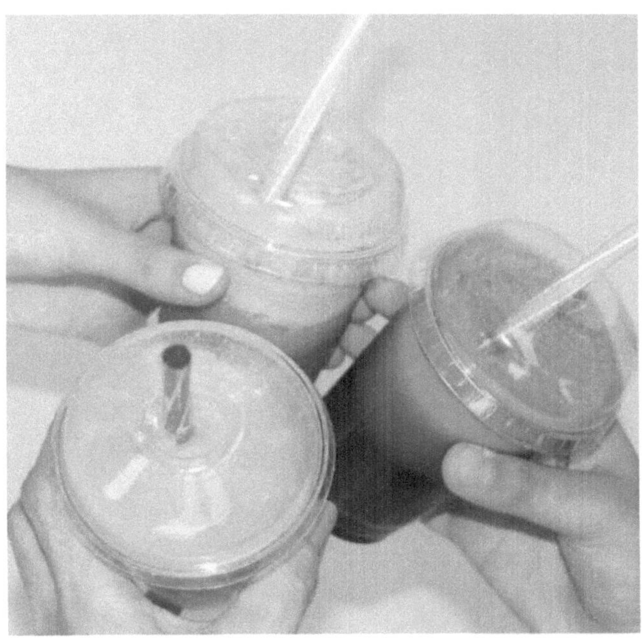

- 1 pomegranate with seeds and white inner skin
- 1 and ½ cup radicchio or substitute with red cabbage
- 20 g flaxseed
- 1 tsp ground turmeric
- Pinch of black pepper
- ½ Tbsp coconut oil
- ¼ tsp ground cinnamon
- Ice

Blend all ingredients in a blender until creamy.

CARROT CUCUMBER SMOOTHIE

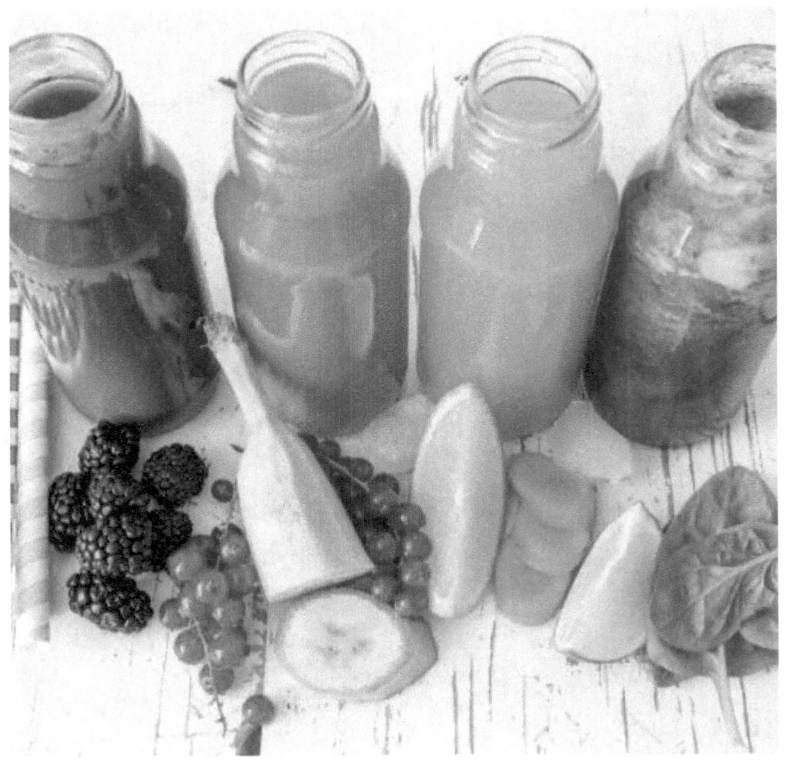

- 1 cucumber
- 2 carrots
- 1 tsp parsley
- Juice of ½ a lemon
- 1 cup water

Blend all ingredients in a blender until creamy.

GREEN PINEAPPLE ORANGE SMOOTHIE

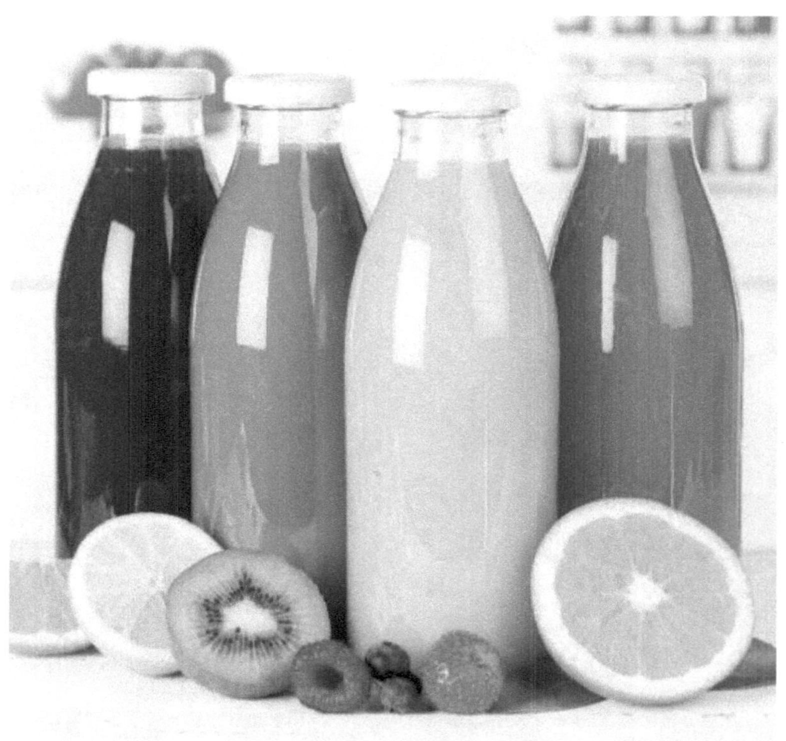

- 1 cup pineapples
- 1 orange, peeled and sliced
- 1 leaf of kale, sliced
- 1 cup coconut milk

- Ice

Blend all ingredients in a blender until creamy.

GREEN APPLE CLEANSE SMOOTHIE

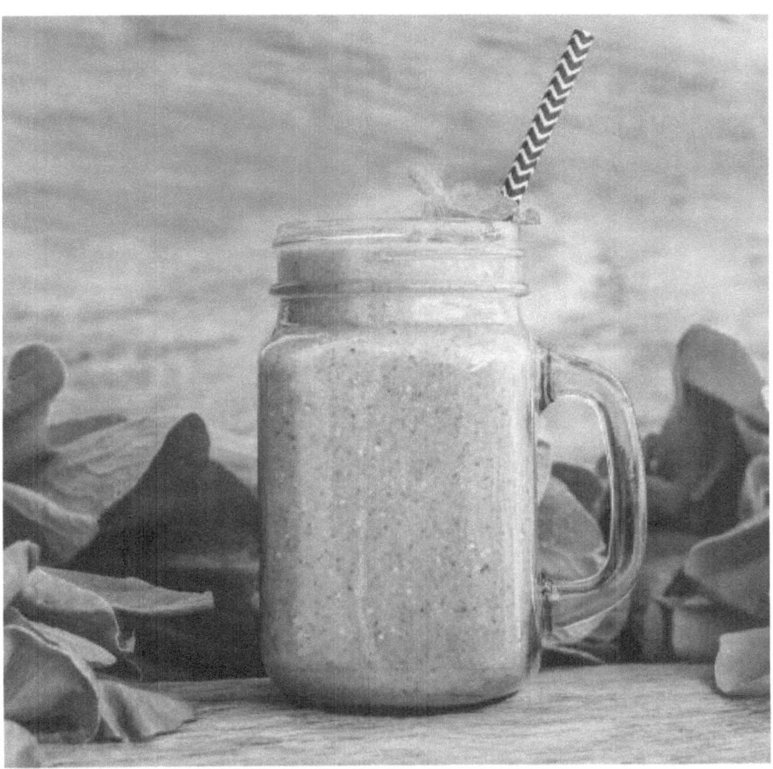

- 1 green apple, sliced and cored, but with skin

- Some spinach leaves or kale
- Juice of ½ lemon
- 1 cucumber, without seeds, sliced, and with skin on
- Some water
- Ice

Blend all ingredients in a blender until creamy.

PINEAPPLE GREEN APPLE CLEANSING SMOOTHIE

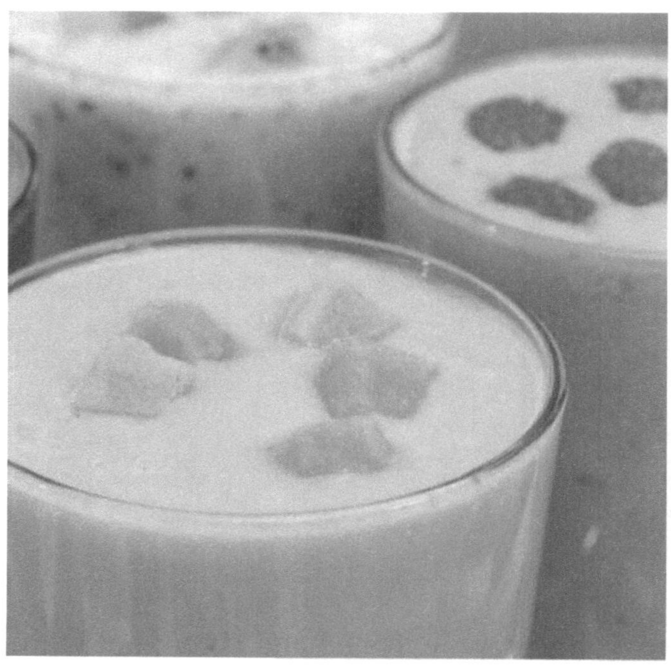

- 1 green apple, cored, sliced but with skin on
- 1 cup pineapple, sliced
- 1 cucumber sliced with skin on
- Some water
- Ice

Blend all ingredients in a blender until creamy.

STRAWBERRY BLUEBERRY CHIA SMOOTHIE

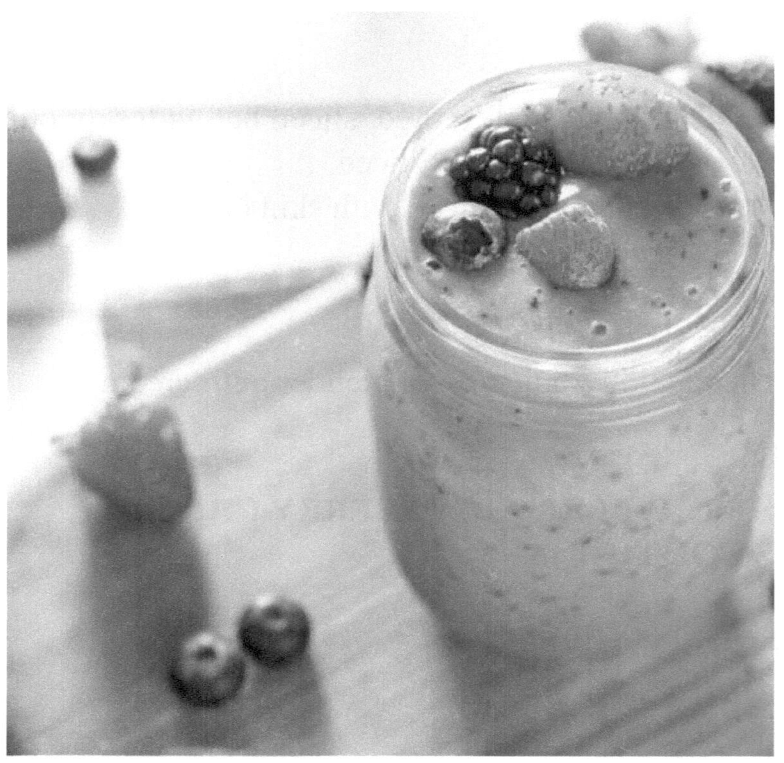

- 1 cup of strawberries sliced
- ½ cup of blueberries
- 1 cup of almond, walnut or rice milk
- ¼ cup of chia seeds
- ¼ cup of fresh mint leaves

Blend all ingredients in a blender until creamy.

MELON GRAPE SMOOTHIE

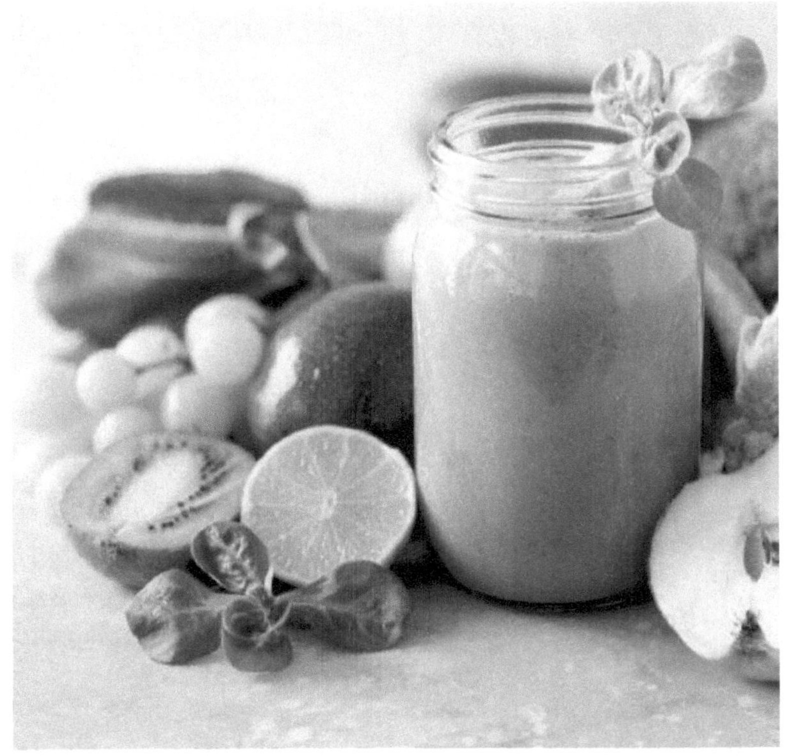

- ¼ cup of green grapes
- ½ cup of melons, cubed
- 1 cup water
- Ice

Blend all ingredients in a blender until creamy.

PARSLEY CABBAGE SMOOTHIE

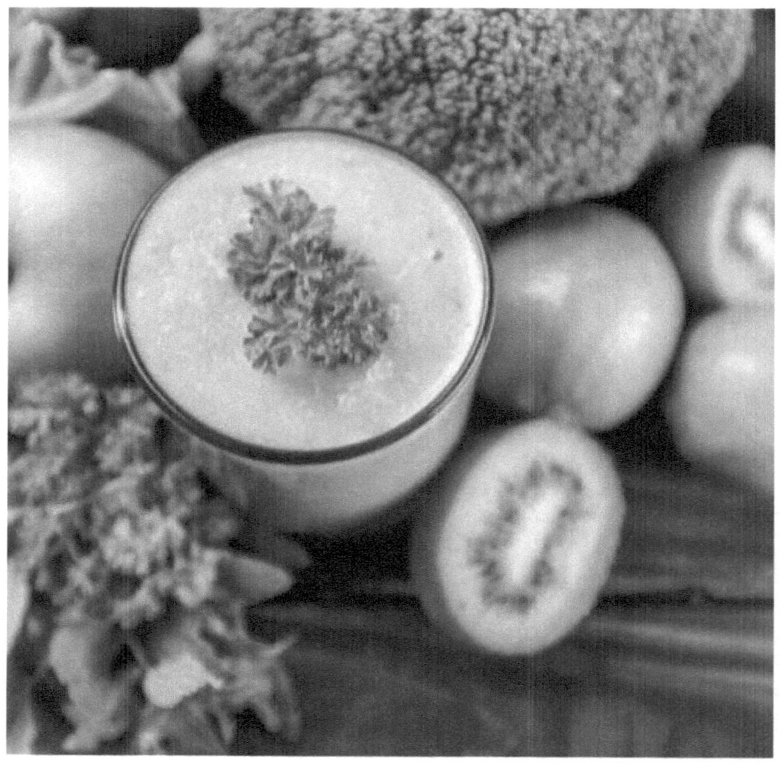

- ½ cup of parsley leaves
- ½ cup of peeled and sliced carrots
- ½ cup of kale, washed and sliced
- Some water

Blend all ingredients in a blender until creamy.

BROCCOLI TOMATOES CELERY SMOOTHIE

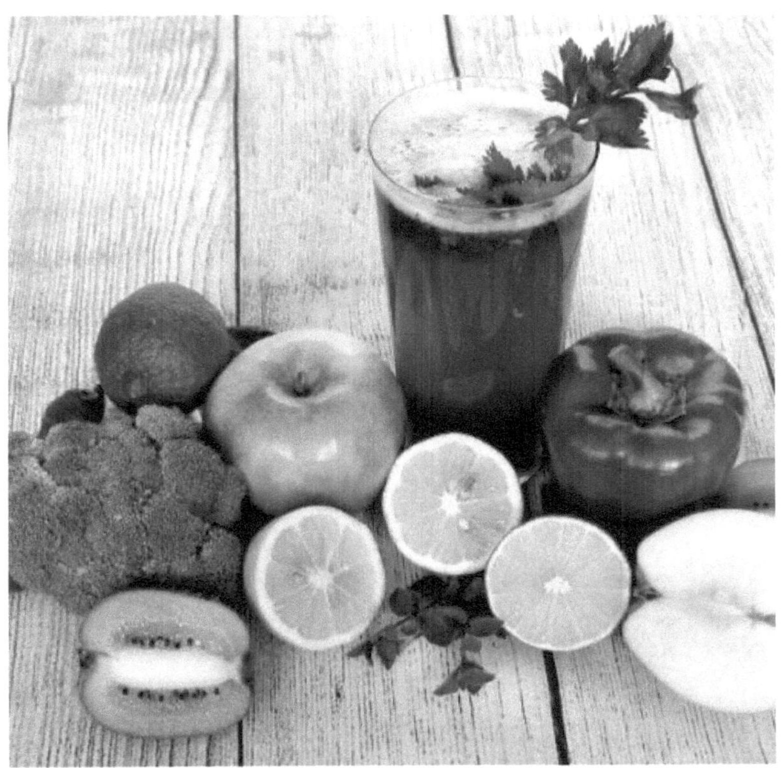

- 150 grams of broccoli flowers
- 2 tomatoes, cubed
- ½ cup of celery sticks

- Water
- Garlic cloves

Blend all ingredients in a blender until creamy.

RADISH CARROT SMOOTHIE

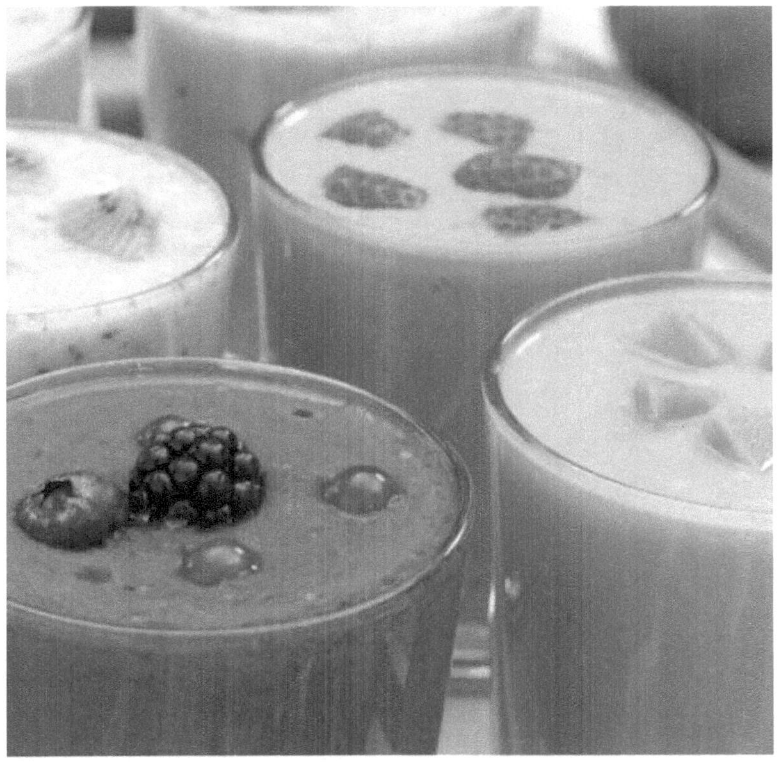

- 1 cup sliced carrots
- 1 cup of sliced radishes
- Water
- Ice

Blend all ingredients in a blender until creamy.

GREEN PEAR SMOOTHIE

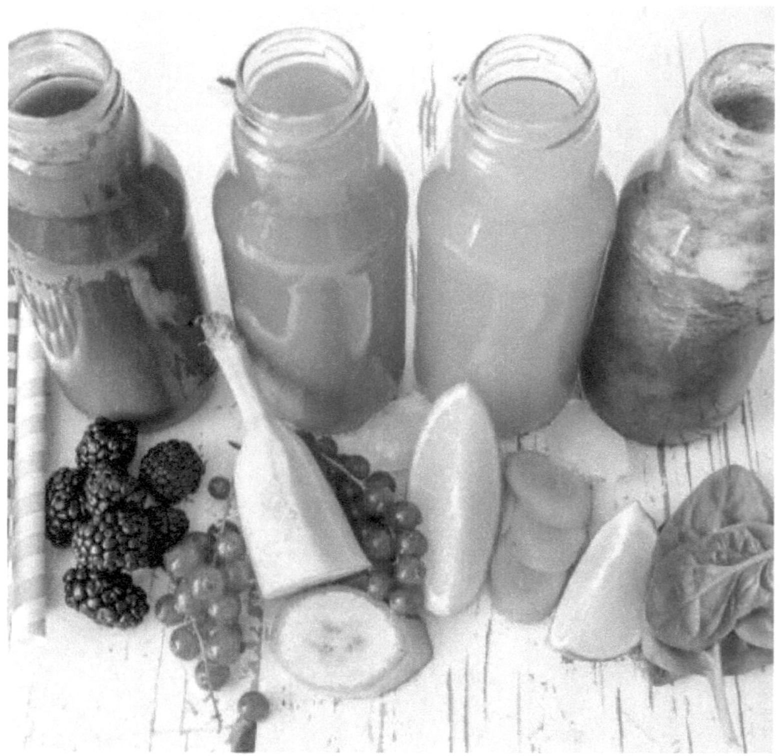

- 2 washed and sliced pears without seeds
- 1cup chopped spinach
- Water
- Ice

Blend all ingredients in a blender until creamy.

APPLE CARROTS SMOOTHIE

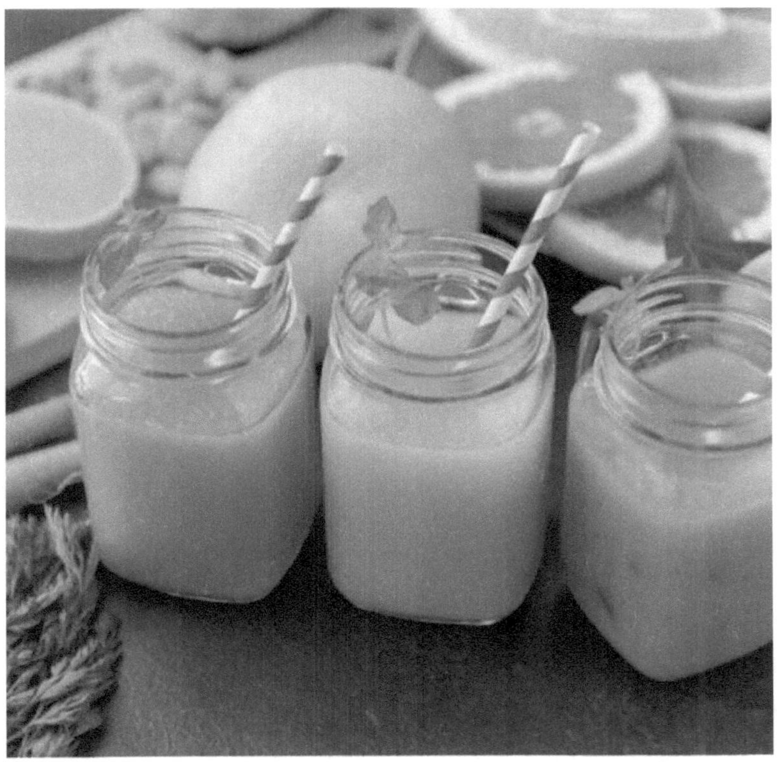

- 1 cup of carrots
- ½ cup red apples, cored and sliced with skin on
- ½ cup green grapes
- 1 orange, peeled, with seeds removed

- Water
- Ice

Blend all ingredients in a blender until creamy.

RED FRUITS AND VEGETABLES LIVER CLEANSE SMOOTHIE

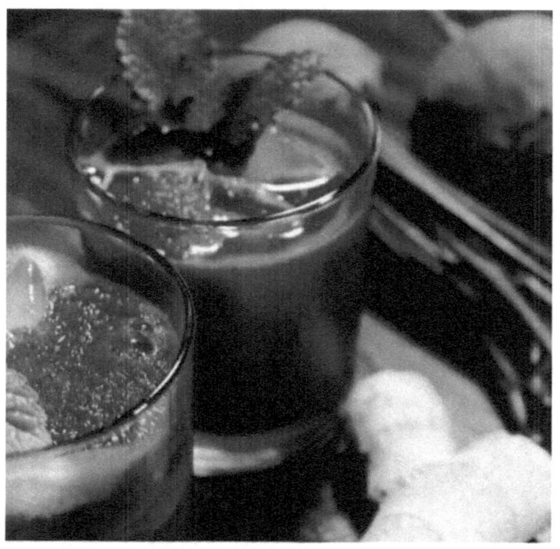

- 1 cup of fresh raw beets
- 1 cup fresh chopped apples
- ½ cup raw chopped carrots
- ¼ cup raw ginger
- ¼ cup flaxseeds
- Handful of parsley leaves
- 1 Tbsp hemp seed oil or flaxseed oil

- Water

Blend all ingredients in a blender until creamy.

BANANA APPLE LIVER CLEANSE SMOOTHIE

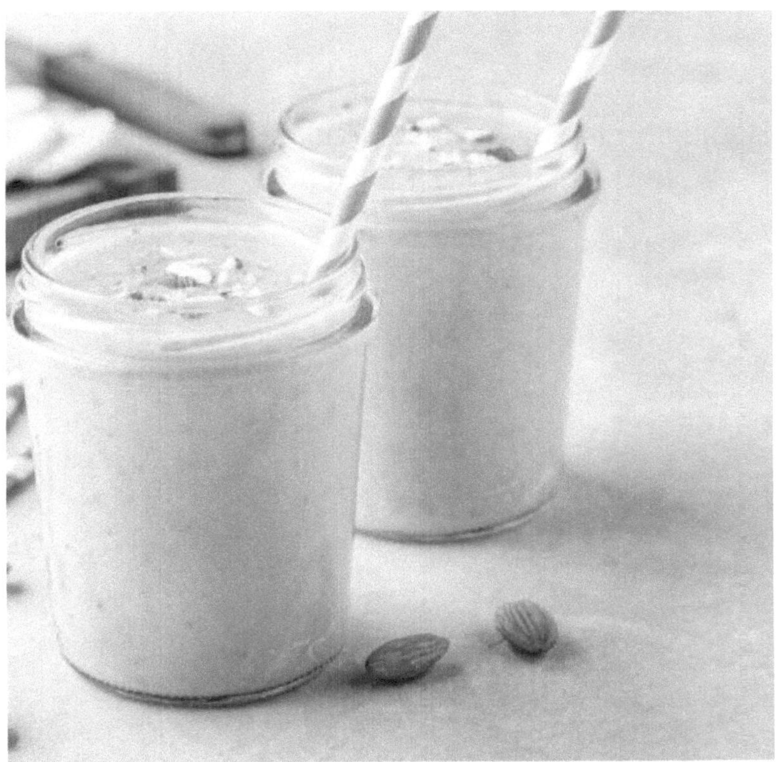

- ½ a banana peeled and sliced
- ½ green apple chopped
- Handful of baby spinach
- ¼ peeled turmeric nub
- 1 Tbsp fresh parsley
- 3 halves walnuts
- 1 Tbsp hemp protein powder
- ½ lemon juiced
- 1 pinch of cinnamon
- ¾ cup almond milk

Blend all ingredients in a blender until creamy.

PINEAPPLE PROTEIN SMOOTHIE

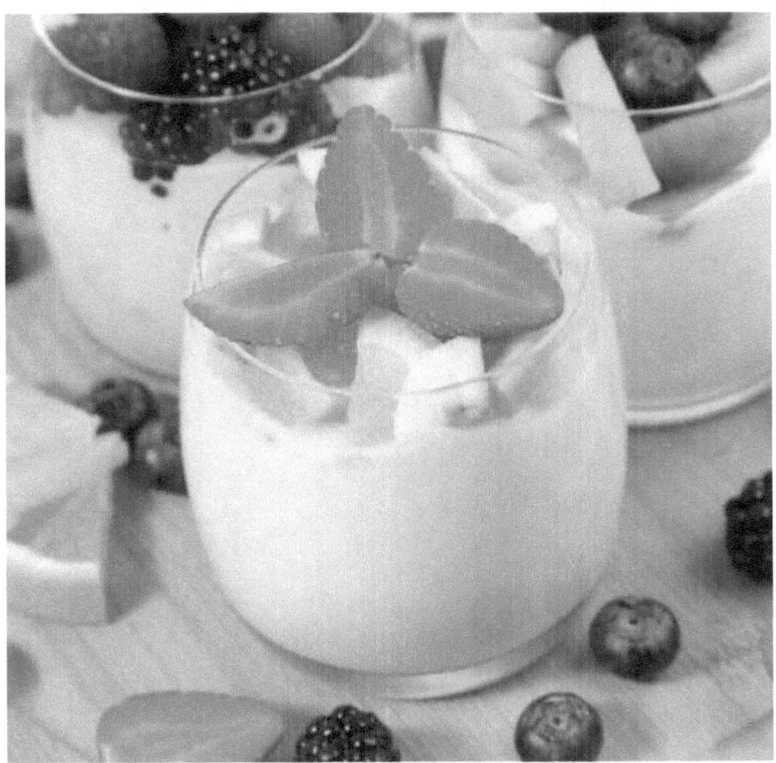

- ¾ cup pineapple sherbet
- 1 scoop vanilla flavored protein whey
- ½ cup water
- 2 ice cubes

Blend all ingredients in a blender until creamy.

CRANBERRY ENERGY SMOOTHIE

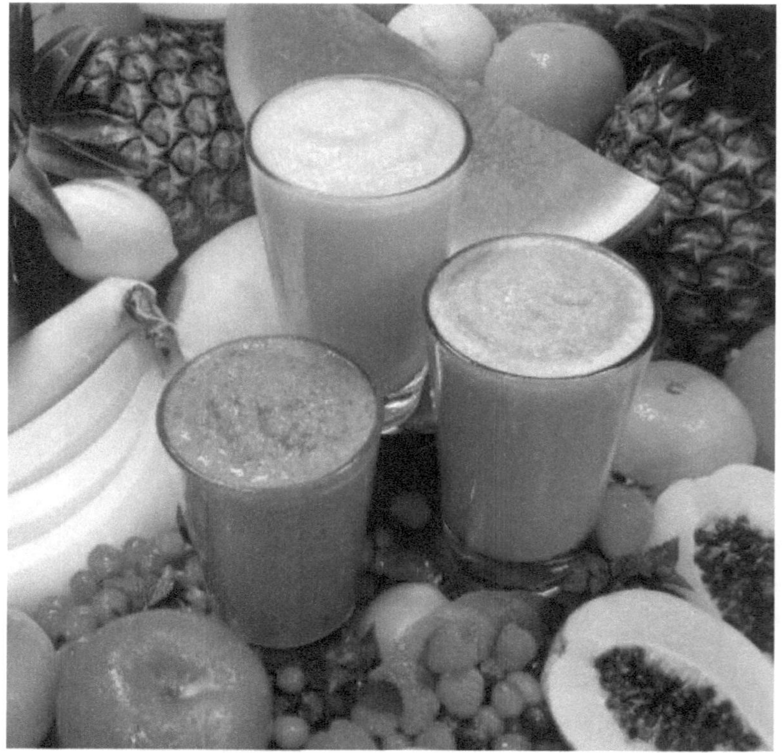

- 1 cup frozen cranberries
- 1 medium cucumber, peeled and sliced
- 1 celery stalk
- 1 handful of parsley
- Squeeze of lime juice

Blend all ingredients in a blender until creamy.

MINTY BLUE SMOOTHIE

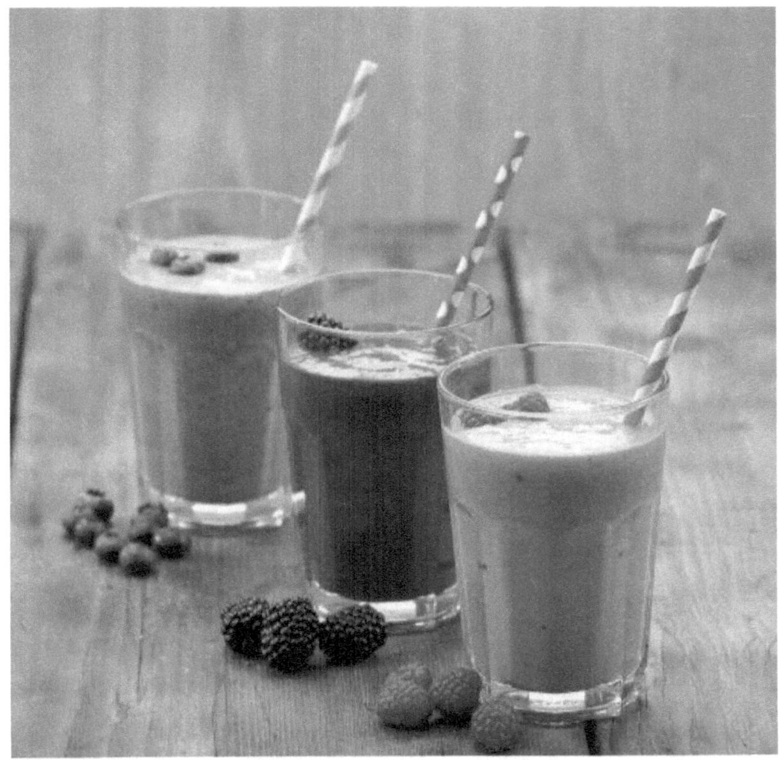

- 1/4 cup frozen blueberries
- 1 sprig of mint leaves
- 1 Tbsp raw honey or stevia

- 1 cup of rice milk
- Ice

Blend all ingredients in a blender until creamy.

SUMMER WATERMELON SMOOTHIE

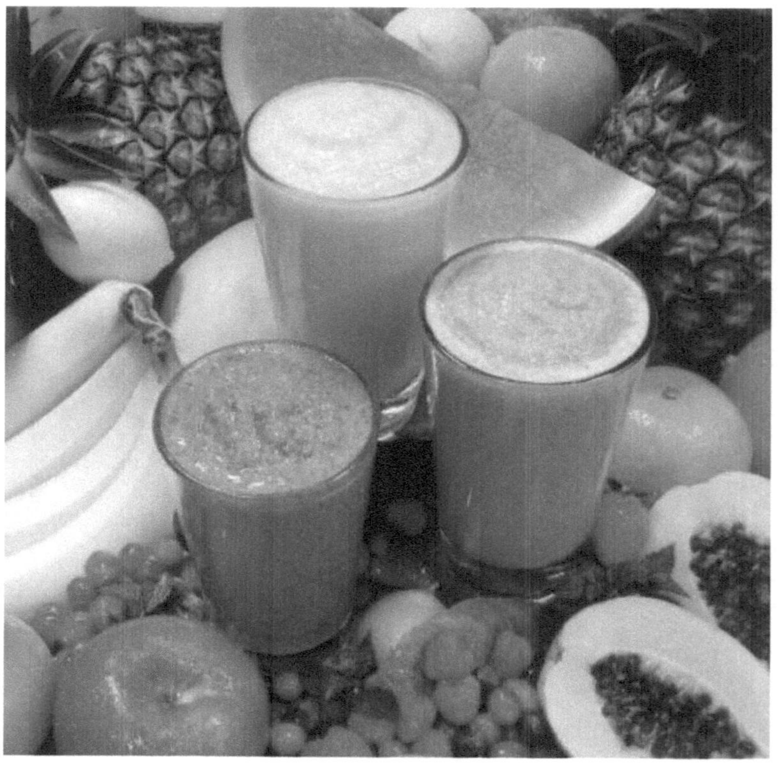

- 1 cup of watermelon cubes, seedless
- 1 tsp lime juice

- 1 Tbsp honey or stevia
- 1 cup ice

Blend all ingredients in a blender until creamy.

STRAWBERRIES APPLE PIE SMOOTHIE

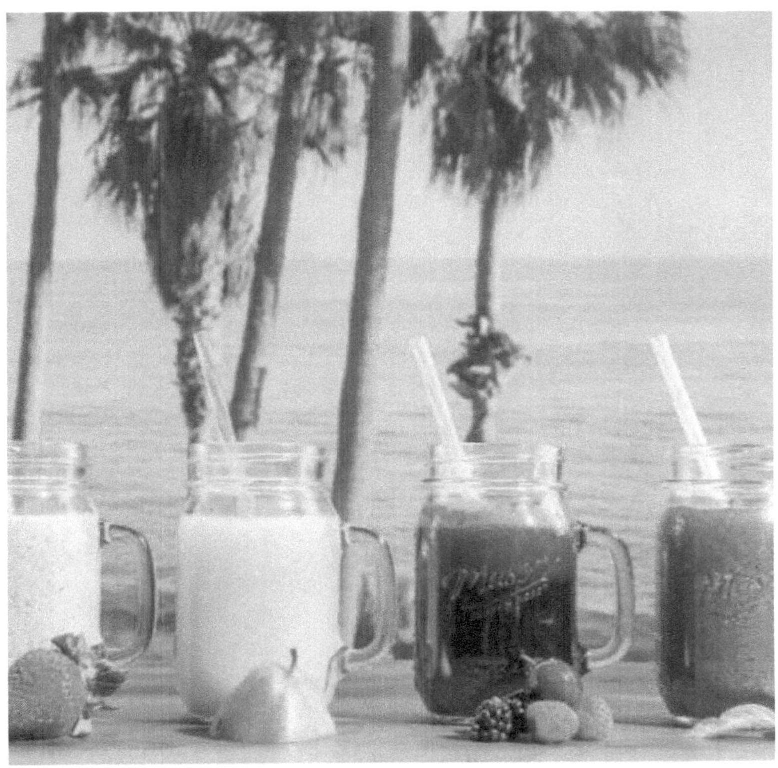

- ½ cup of strawberries

- ½ cup unsweetened applesauce
- ½ cup plain yogurt
- ¼ cup rice milk
- ½ Tbsp oat or wheat bran

Blend all ingredients in a blender until creamy.

3 BERRIES SMOOTHIE

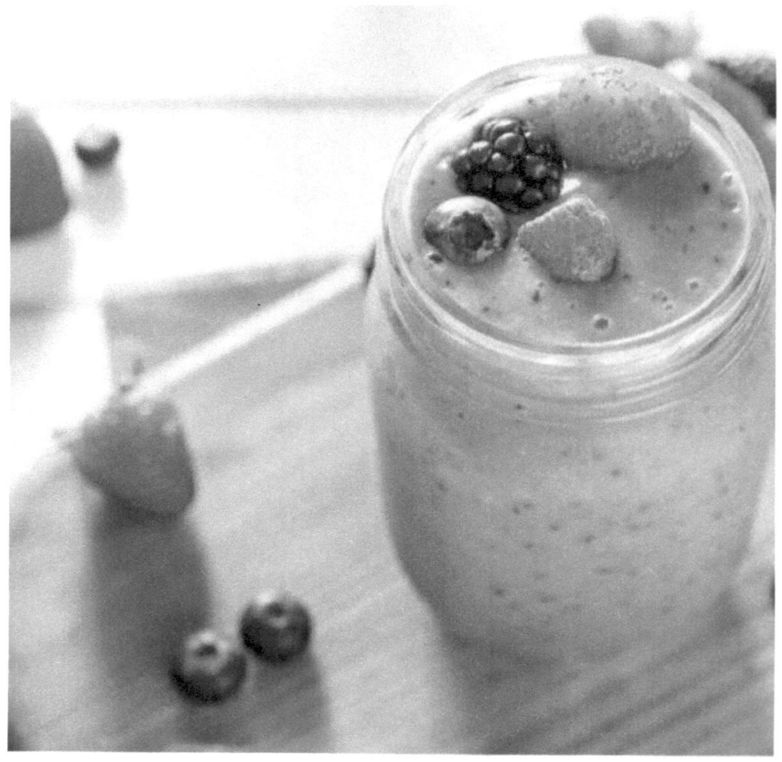

- ½ cup frozen unsweetened raspberries
- ½ cup frozen unsweetened blueberries
- ¼ cup unsweetened cranberry juice
- 2/3 cup silken firm tofu
- 1 tsp vanilla extract

Blend all ingredients in a blender until creamy.

COCONUT PINEAPPLE SMOOTHIE

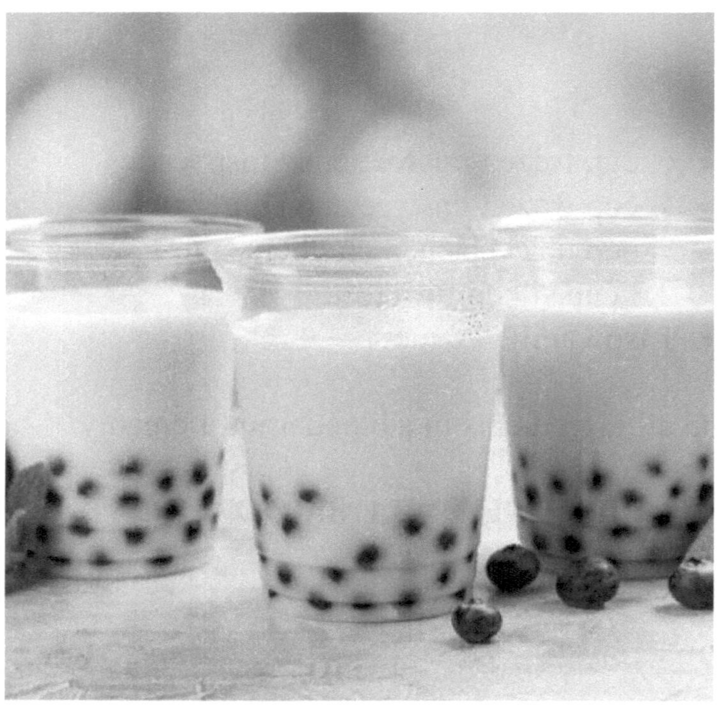

- 2 cups of pineapple chunks
- 1 can coconut milk unsweetened
- 1 cup almond milk unsweetened
- 1 tsp turmeric
- 1 Tbsp grated ginger

Blend all ingredients in a blender until creamy.

STRAWBERRY CHEESECAKE SMOOTHIE

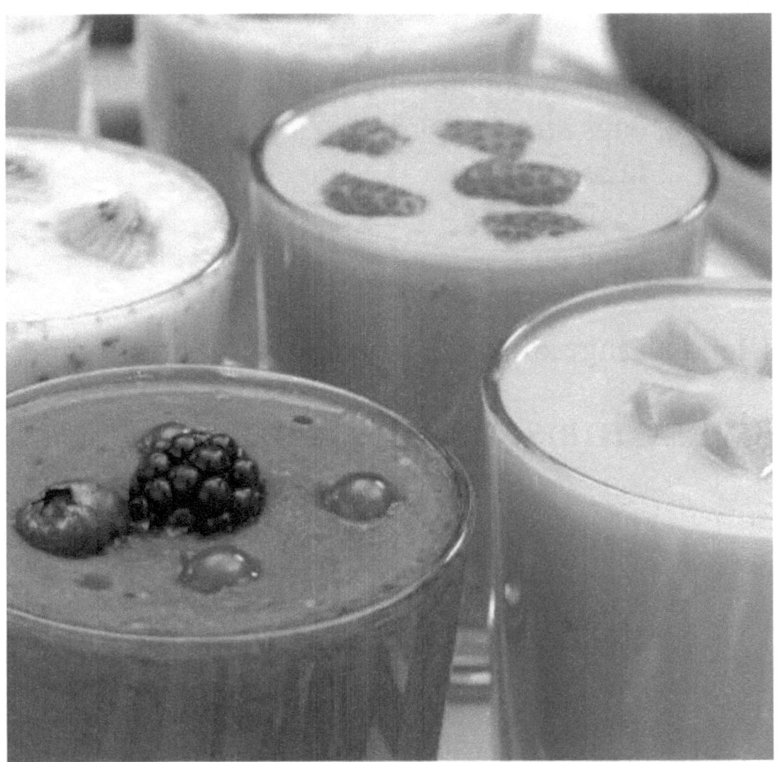

- 1 cup of strawberries, hulled
- 1 cup unsweetened rice milk
- 2 Tbsp cream cheese softened
- 1 tsp vanilla extract
- ½ tsp honey

- 3 to 4 ice cubes

Blend all ingredients in a blender until creamy.

WATERMELON STRAWBERRY

- 4 cups of cubed watermelon
- 2 cups strawberries
- 2 limes, peeled
- 2 basil leaves
- 2 cups ice

Blend all ingredients in a blender until creamy.

SWEET HIBISCUS SMOOTHIE

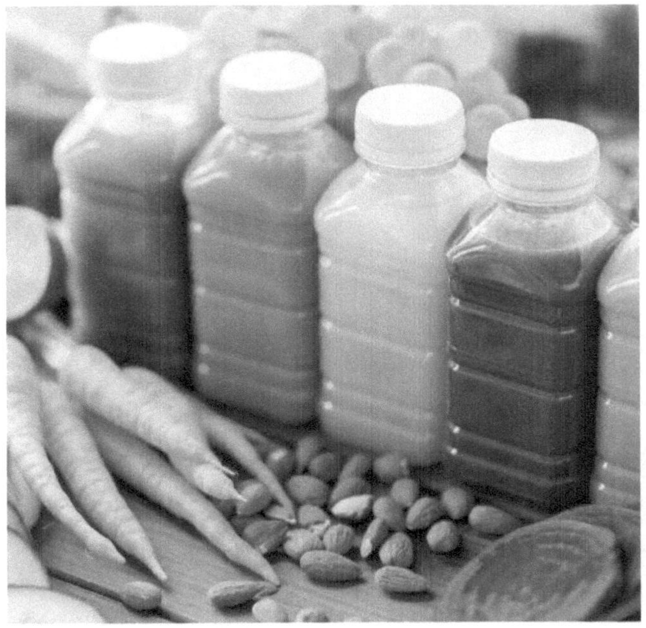

- ¼ cup dried hibiscus petals
- 8 cups water
- ¼ cups maple syrup
- 2 Tbsp grated ginger
- 2 limes juiced
- Ice

Put ginger, maple syrup and hibiscus petals into a pot with the water and bring to a broil. Let cool and add to a blender with ice. Add lime juice. Blend all ingredients in a blender until creamy.

COCONUT COFFEE SMOOTHIE

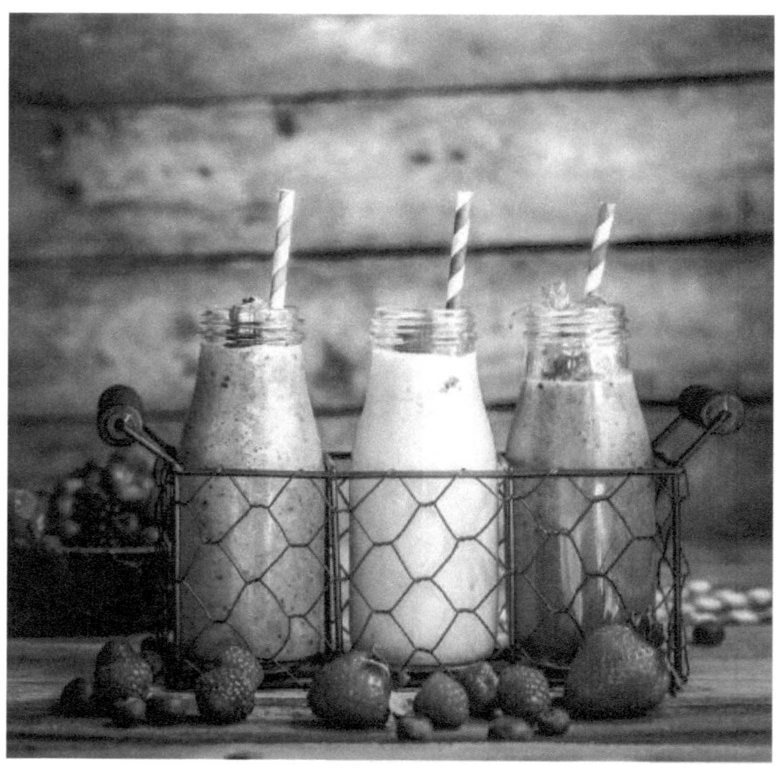

- ¾ cup coffee brewed
- ½ cup coconut milk unsweetened
- ¼ cup ice
- ¼ tsp cinnamon
- 2 tsp maple syrup

Blend all ingredients in a blender until creamy.

SPICY PAPAYA SMOOTHIE

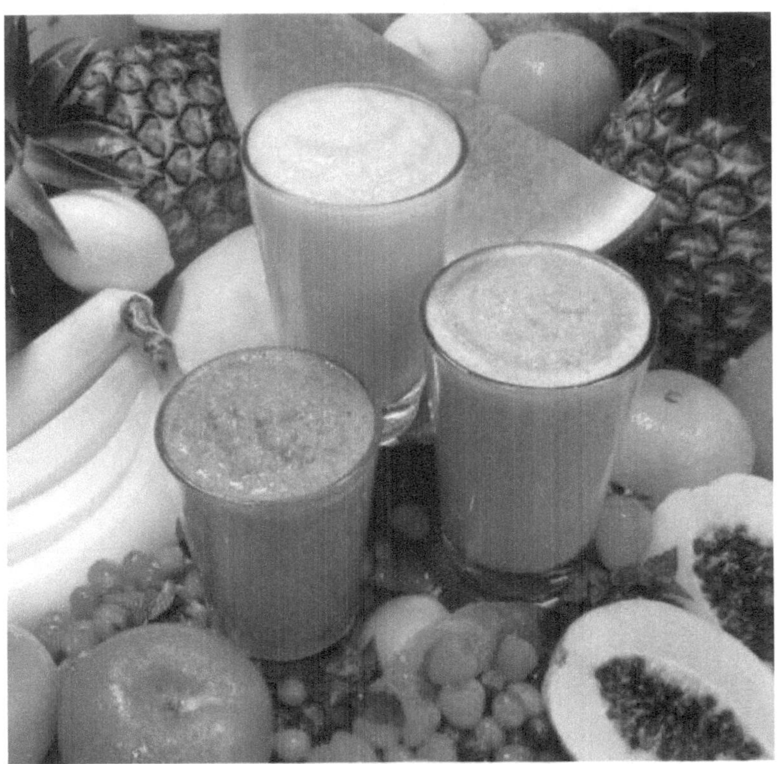

- ½ papaya cut in slices
- ½ cup almond milk
- 1 tsp honey
- ½ tsp grated ginger
- 2 Tbspn lime juice

Blend all ingredients in a blender until creamy.

WATERMELON KIWI SMOOTHIE

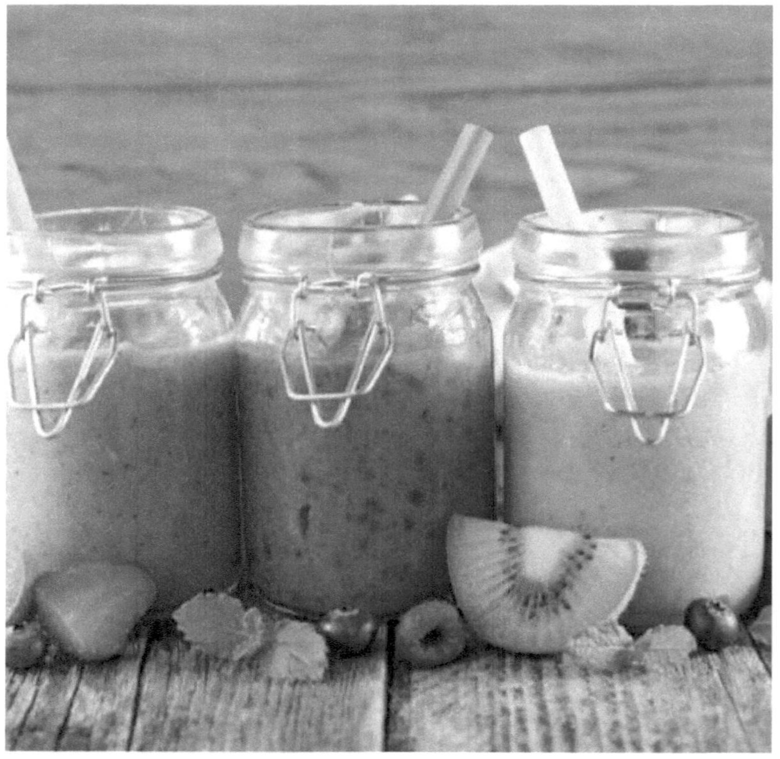

- 2 cups watermelon chunks
- 1 peeled kiwifruit
- 1 cup ice

Blend all ingredients in a blender until creamy.

COLD-BREW ICED GREEN TEA

- 6 cups of water at room temperature
- 4 green tea bags
- 2 or 3 lemon slices

Combine all ingredients in a pitcher or large container with a lid and refrigerate for at least 8 hours. Remove the tea bags, straining the liquid. Discard the tea bags and lemon slices. Sweeten as desired, stirring well. Chill until ready to serve over ice.

CHAI CONCENTRATE

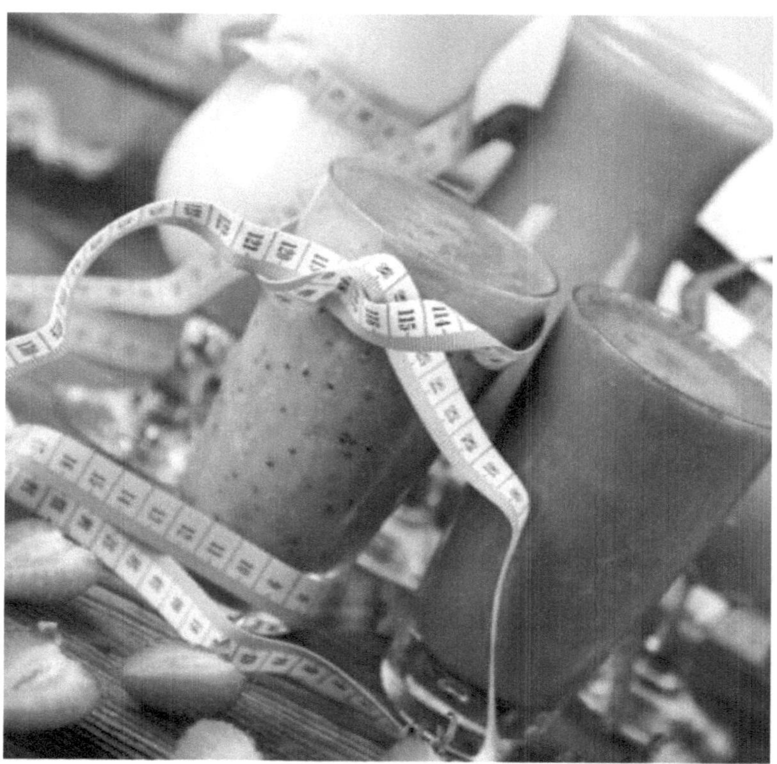

- 20 black peppercorns
- 8 cardamom pods
- 10 cloves
- 2 cinnamon sticks
- 4 cups water
- 1 (2-inch) sliced fresh ginger
- 4 black tea bags

- 2 tablespoons maple syrup or honey
- ¼ teaspoon pure vanilla extract
- Dairy or nondairy milk for serving

Put peppercorns, cardamom, cloves, and cinnamon in a medium saucepan and cook over medium, stirring frequently, for 3 or 4 minutes until fragrant and lightly golden. Add water and ginger, bring to a boil. Reduce the heat to medium-low; simmer, partially covered, for 10 minutes. Remove from the heat and add tea bags and steep for 5 minutes. Remove the tea bags, gently squeezing them to release excess water before discarding the bags.

Add the maple syrup and vanilla. Stil to combine. Let stand for 1 hour; strain and discard the solids. Store the concentrate in an airtight container in the refrigerator for up to 1 week. To prepare, combine ½ to ¾ cup milk with 1 cup concentrate. Serve hot or cold over ice.

GOJI BERRIES DATES SMOOTHIE

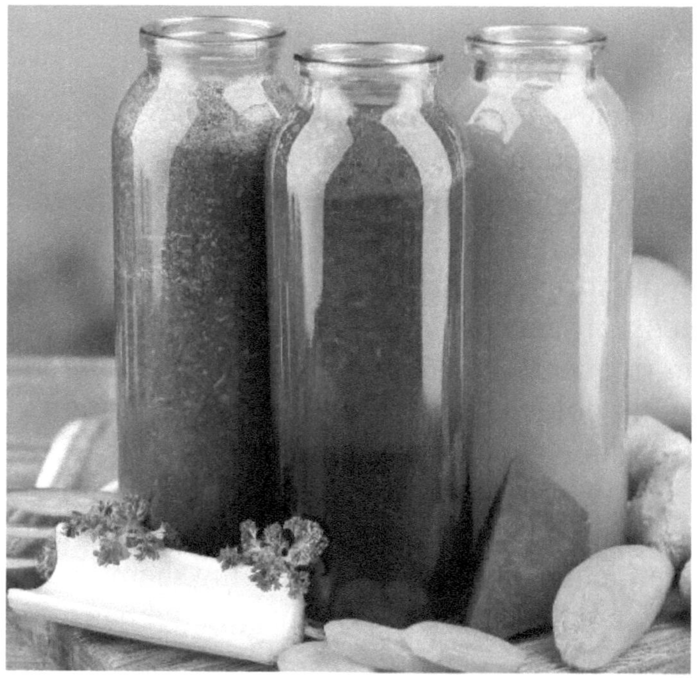

- Water
- Goji Berries
- Dates
- Ice

Put Goji Berries in pitcher.
Pour cold or warm water on Berries.
Steep until the water turns a lovely reddish color and the Goji's are plump. This will be a shorter amount of time if it's warm water versus cold water.

Add dates and ice. Blend in blender until creamy.

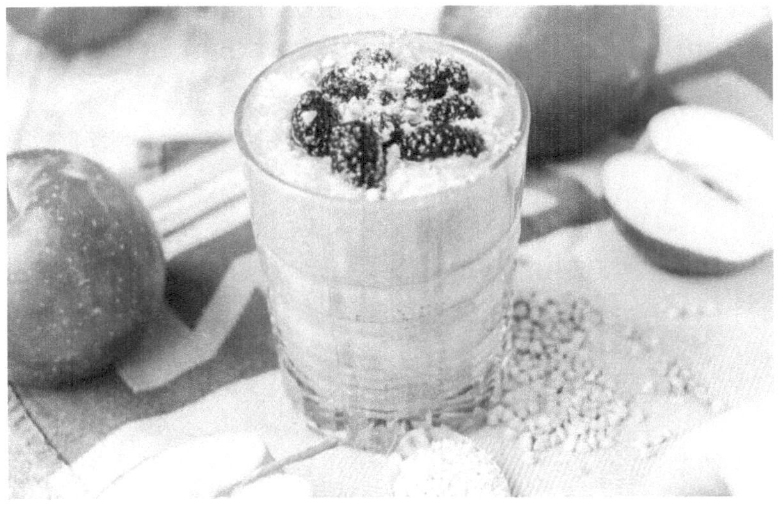

SPIRULLINA APPLES BERRIES SMOOTHIE

- 3 Granny Smith apples
- 2 bananas
- ¼ cup pitted dates
- ¼ cup cashews
- ½ tsp cinnamon
- Coupons
- 1 tbs spirulina

- 1 cup water
- Ice as desired

Core the apples and peel the bananas.
Add all ingredients into a high-speed blender.
Blend on a high speed for approximately 1 minute,
or until all ingredients are broken down.
Serve immediately.

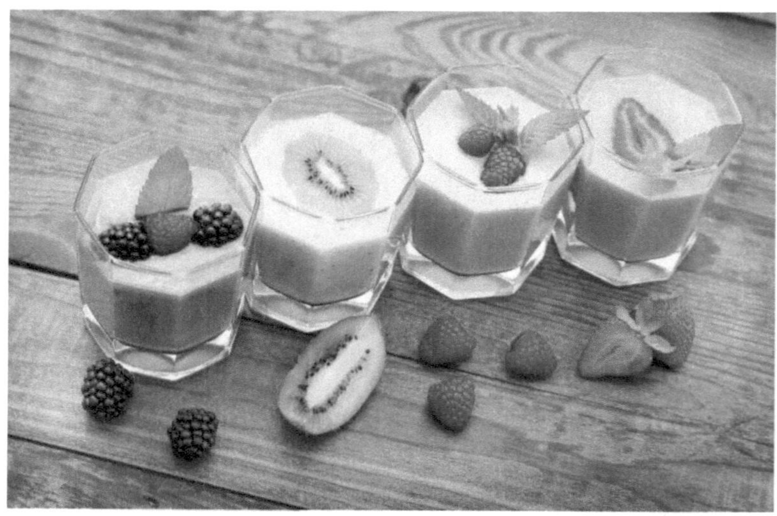

STRAWBERRY KIWI BLACKBERRY SMOOTHIES

- 1 banana
- 6 strawberries
- 1 kiwi
- 1/2 cup vanilla frozen yogurt
- 3/4 cup pineapple and orange juice blend

Place the banana, strawberries, kiwi, vanilla frozen yogurt, and pineapple and orange juice blend in a blender. Blend until smooth.

Or make separate smoothies for each fruit by placing 1 fruit with yogurt and juice then blend.

BERRIES VANILLA SMOOTHIE

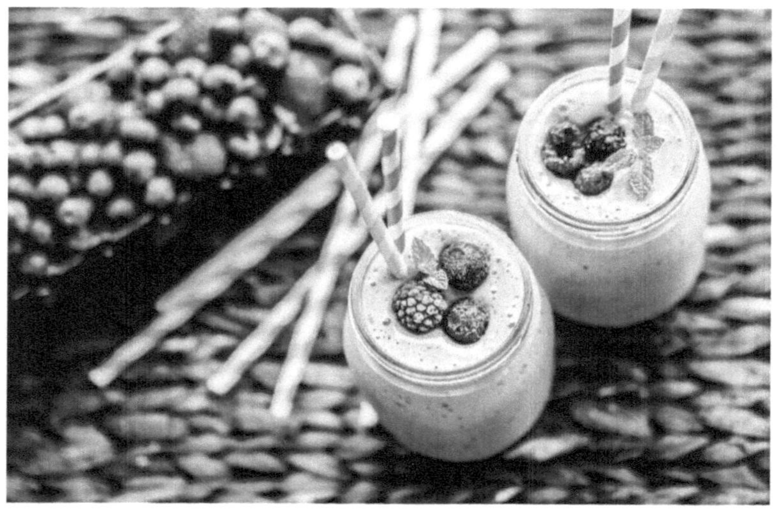

- ½ medium banana sliced into ½ inches and frozen
- 4 ounces of frozen unsweetened berries
- 1 container (6 ounces) fat-free vanilla yogurt
- ½ cup fat-free milk
- ¼ teaspoon vanilla extract

Put everything into a blender and process for 30 seconds until thick and smooth.

FRENCH VANILLA ICED CAFFE LATTE

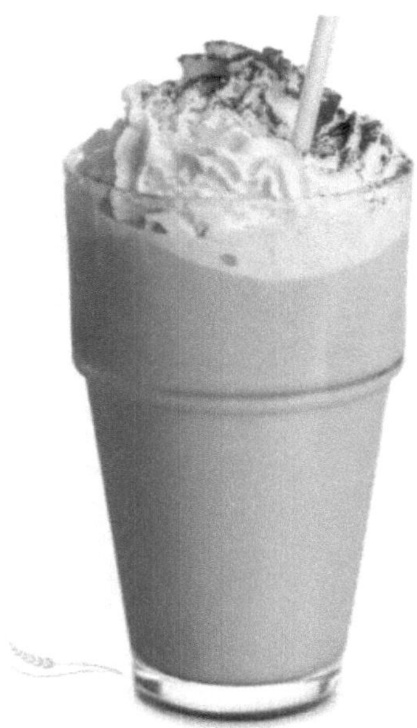

- 6 cups of strong coffee (decaf or regular)
- 2 tablespoons Stevia sweetener
- 2 cups of fat-free French Vanilla creamer
- Skim milk

Pour all ingredients into a pitcher, refrigerate, and serve over ice.

ORANGE-STRAWBERRY FROTHIN' AT THE MOUTHIN'

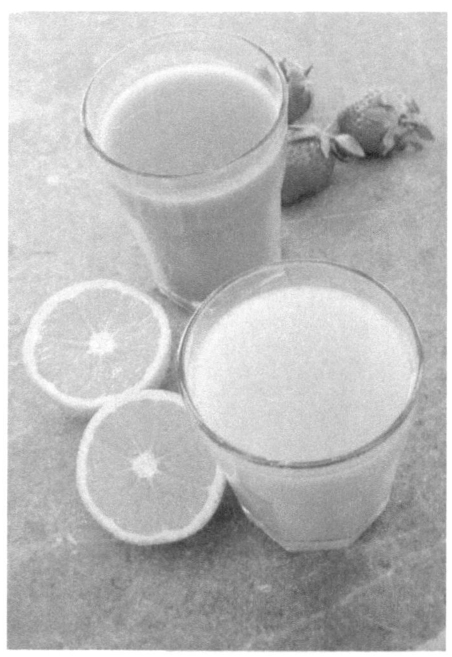

- 2 cups fresh orange juice
- 1 ½ cups apricot nectar
- 1 cup frozen unsweetened strawberries

Blend everything in a blender until smooth and frothy.

REFRESHING LIMEADE

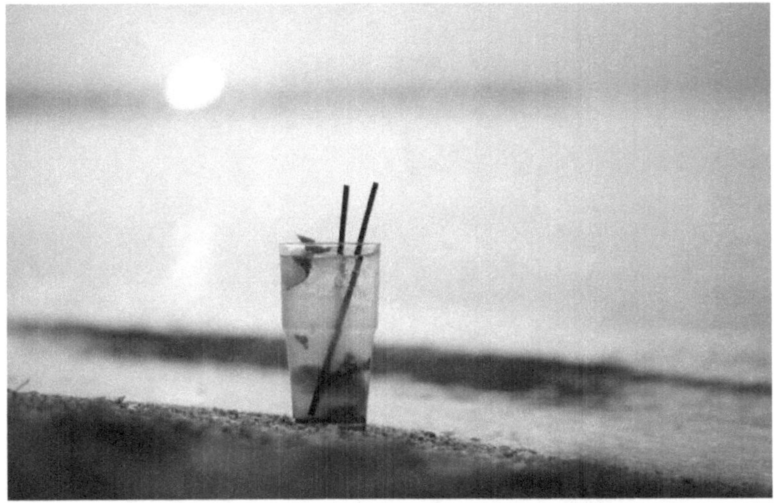

- 5¼ cups water
- ¼ cup Stevia sweetener
- Lime zest
- Lemon zest
- Lemon Juice (3 lemons)
- Lime Juice (3 limes)
- Ice

In a small saucepan, boil water with ¼ cup of the water, add the Stevia sweetener and stir until dissolved. Remove the pan from the heat and stir in the zest from lemon and lime, the juice. Add 5 cups of cold water to the mixture and add ice.

Kailin Gow

MOONLIGHT MOCHA CAPPUCCINO

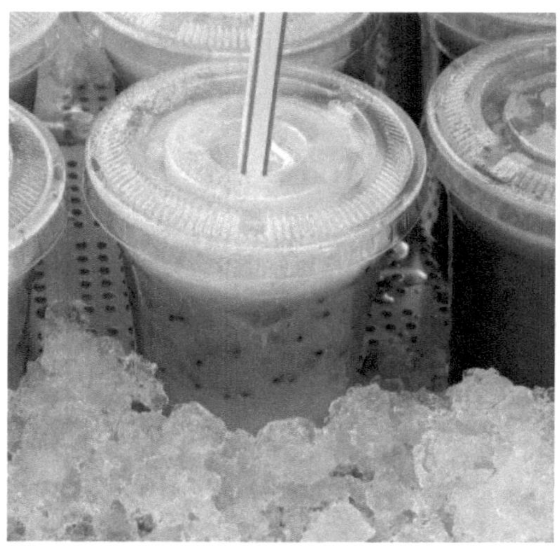

- 2 cups fat-free milk or plant-base unsweetened milk alternative
- 1 ½ cups strong hot dark roast coffee (can be decaf or regular)

Heat the milk in a microwave-safe cup and pour into a blender with the hot coffee. Blend on high speed for 1 minute. Pour into separate coffee mugs and stir in the syrup and Stevia sweetener. Top with non-fat whipped topping and sprinkle with cocoa powder. Add crescent or star-shaped sprinkles for a moonlight effect.

REFRESHING RASPBERRY TEA SPRITZER

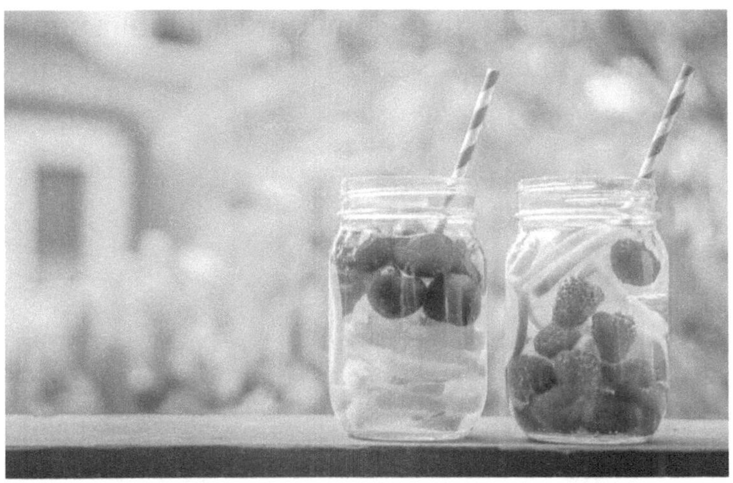

- 1 cup water
- 2 bag green tea
- 2 teaspoons honey
- ¼ teaspoon fresh lemon juice
- ½ cup frozen unsweetened raspberries
- ¾ cup chilled sparkling water

Boil some water in a pan. Pour into a glass measuring cup, add the tea bag and steep for 4 minutes and discard the bag. Stir in honey and lemon juice. Cool down the tea mixture in the glass cup by placing the cup in a container filled with cold ice water. Let sit until the tea mixture is room temperature. In a blender pour the tea mixture in along with the raspberries, blend, and strain the mixture, removing the seeds. Pour the sparkling water into the tea mixture and pour into tall ice-filled glasses. Serve!

*****

About the Author

Kailin Gow is an award-winning USA Today Bestselling author of over 700 books, tv host, award-winning filmmaker, mom, and humanitarian. She has traveled to over 50 countries, taken cooking lessons from top chefs, and grew up in the hospitality industry as a hotelier and restauranteur. She lives in the American West, and is always on the go!

Want to Know More about *ways to improve your life, live more fully, tips on finance, health, travel, relationships, and more*?

Sign Up for Kailin's Free Go Girl Newsletter at:

http://www.subscribepage.com/g9r7j6